Cannabis
and CBD
Science
for Dogs

Natural Supplements to Support Healthy Living and Graceful Aging

D. Caroline Coile, Ph.D.

ASSISI BIO PRESS

978-0-9976607-0-8 (Paperback)
978-0-9976607-1-5 (eBook)

Published by Assisi Bio Press
publisher@AssisiBioPress.org

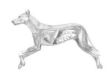

TABLE OF CONTENTS

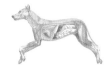

PREFACE

My background is in science. My Ph.D. is in experimental psychology and neuroscience. I like Western medicine. I don't do crystals or reiki or faith healing or homeopathy. I am skeptical of acupuncture but concede it probably has its place. I tried it with my dogs twice, and it didn't work, so I think its place is not with me. Show me auras and feelings and energy fields, and I remain unconvinced when it comes to medicine. Show me chemicals and neurotransmitters and data points, and I'm listening.

So when I heard about medical cannabis for pets, I was skeptical. It sounded a little too much like a New Age touchy-feely "a stoned dog is a happy dog" approach for me.

For starters, there was the credulity-begging long and diverse list of claims: antianxiety, antiseizure, anti-inflammatory, antibacterial—what was next? Anticancer? Oh yeah, antitumor also on the list. That sounded suspiciously like snake oil to me.

But there's a fine line between being skeptical and closed-minded, so I (grudgingly) decided to read some of the science (and at that point I was using the term loosely) before shutting my mind to it.

I was about to get an education. First, medical cannabis isn't about getting stoned. Medical cannabis for pets doesn't even have significant THC in it. "What a scam!" I thought. "What's the good of hemp without THC?" Then I learned that THC is far from the only significant cannabinoid in cannabis, and that in fact another, cannabidiol (CBD), is the one that seems to be providing the greatest health benefits. And cannabidiol has no psychoactive effects. So much for stoned dogs lounging around the house.

The more I delved into the subject, the more I found that this was no esoteric fringe science, but a robust area of research. One peer-reviewed paper after another presented data that supported health benefits of cannabinoids—some tentatively, some convincingly. That long list of claims? It turns out there's a valid scientific reason for it: cannabinoid receptors are literally all over the body, acting as homeostatic directors of myriad other neurotransmitters.

BUT CAN IT HELP YOUR DOG?

During my research, I conducted many interviews with pet owners. Anecdotal evidence doesn't carry the weight of controlled scientific experimentation, but talking to these people was compelling. In many cases they reported that cannabinoids had saved their dogs' lives, or at least dramatically improved their quality of life.

Do I believe cannabinoids are miracle workers? No. I don't believe any substance can do it all. But I am convinced cannabinoids have some tantalizing and very likely major health benefits.

Which brings me to the big question: Would I give cannabinoids to my own dogs? The short answer is yes. And if you know me, that's a huge turnaround, because my dogs are the center of my world—just as I am sure yours are the center of your world. And we all want what's best for them.

PROCEEDS FROM THIS BOOK

All proceeds from this book are donated to charitable organizations which benefit animal rescue, animal health, veterinary research, and animal welfare. Primary recipients are the **San Diego Humane Society** (www.sdhumane.org/) and the **American Kennel Club Canine Health Foundation** (www.akcchf.org/).

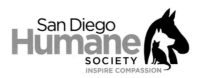

Founded in 1880, the San Diego Humane Society is a private nonprofit providing vital services to animals and people by sheltering and adopting animals, providing positive reinforcement training classes, investigating animal cruelty and neglect, presenting education programs for youth and adults, and much more. As of 2015, San Diego county reached zero euthanasia for healthy and treatable animals, and is the "safest place to be a pet."

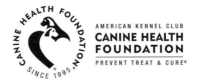

The American Kennel Club Canine Health Foundation is dedicated to advancing the health of all dogs and their owners by funding scientific research and supporting the dissemination of health information to prevent, treat, and cure canine disease. Since 1995, the CHF has become the largest funder of exclusively canine health research in the world.

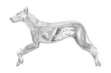

CHAPTER 1:

CANNABIS, HEMP, & MARIJUANA

The indisputable benefits of cannabis for the treatment of a variety of medical conditions have brought about the widespread cultural acceptance of medical marijuana. Not only are people more open to cannabis as a natural therapy, they are also considering this option for their dogs.

This surge of interest has brought to light the general confusion between marijuana and hemp, which involves both legality, chemical composition, and therapeutic application. These differences are especially important when it comes to medical cannabis for pets.

BACKGROUND

Cannabis has been grown for thousands of years for rope, fabric, oils, and foods, for its psychoactive effects for religious purposes, and most significantly for our discussion, for its medical purposes.

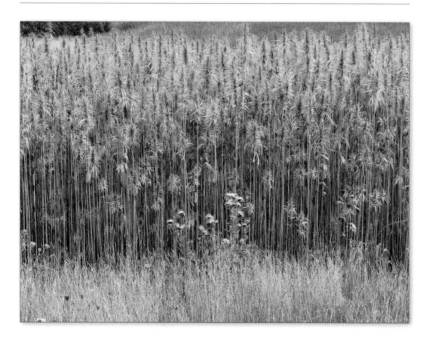

Cannabis has been used as a medicine since ancient times. There is evidence of its use as long ago as 5000 BCE in China and 1000 BCE in India (as mentioned in the sacred Hindu Hymns of Atharvaveda). It was documented by the Greeks in 512 CE in the Vienna Dioscorides.

By the late 1800s it was around the third most commonly used medicine worldwide.

The rest of the world continues to grow and use hemp as an agricultural crop, producing tens of millions of acres of industrial hemp crops and millions of tons of industrial hemp products, many of which are imported into the U.S. and available in health food stores, grocery stores, clothing stores, and more. This crop remains true to the therapeutic and nutritional hemp used by ancient cultures and has safely been incorporated in the global food supply for both people and animals for thousands of years.

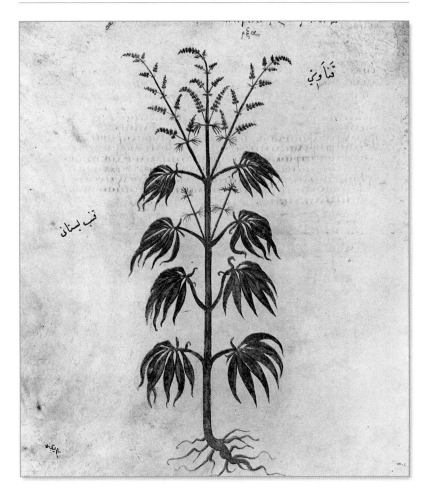

CANNABIS AND HEMP IN AMERICA

The Puritans brought hemp seed with them to colonial America; hemp was used in the lines, sails and caulking of the Mayflower. British sailing vessels always had a store of hemp seed, and Britain's colonies were compelled by law to grow hemp.

By the mid-1600s, hemp had become an important part of the economy in the New World. The colonies produced cordage, cloth, canvas, sacks, and paper from hemp, most of it destined

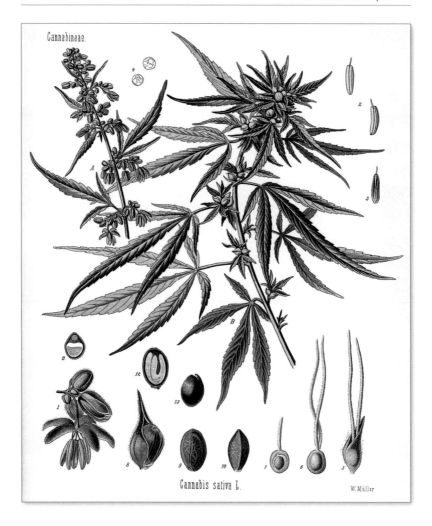

for British consumption. The first drafts of the Declaration of Independence were penned on hemp paper.

In America's early days, farmers were compelled by patriotic duty to grow hemp, and could even pay taxes with it. George Washington encouraged all citizens to sow hemp, as did he. Thomas Jefferson bred improved hemp varieties.

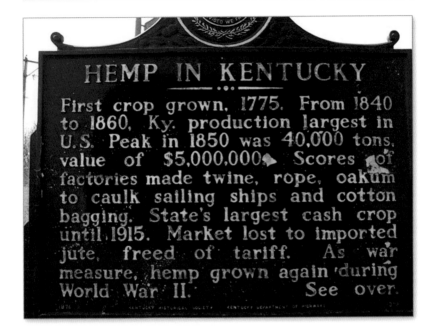

Kentucky, followed by Missouri and Illinois, produced most American hemp until the late 1800s, when demand for sailcloth and cordage began to wane with the decline of sailing ships. From the end of the Civil War until World War I, Kentucky was the only state with a significant hemp industry.

Major American pharmaceutical companies produced many cannabis-based medicines from the mid-1800s to 1937. Initially, medical cannabis was imported from India, but domestic production began in 1913. With World War I thwarting importation, the U.S. became self-sufficient. By 1918, U.S. farmers produced 60,000 pounds annually.[1]

The Marihuana Tax Act of 1937 brought an end to marijuana and hemp cultivation in the U.S., with one final burst during World War II due to the USDA's Hemp for Victory campaign.

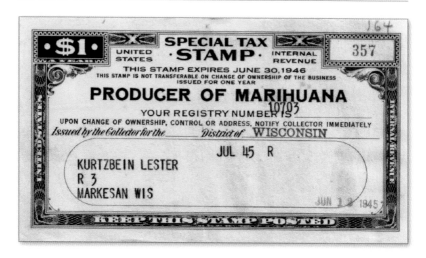

MARIJUANA VS HEMP

Marijuana is the name for forms of cannabis with high levels of THC (once 1-5%, now potentially 30% or more). THC is the dominant cannabinoid (chemical compounds found in cannabis that act on cells in the brain), the psychoactive component of marijuana (what gets people "high"), and the component of cannabis that is regarded as a controlled substance. Most people think THC is also responsible for its medicinal benefits, but that's only part of the story.

Hemp is another form of cannabis, one that has high levels of a non-psychoactive cannabinoid called cannabidiol (CBD) rather than THC. Hemp is the cannabis source used for CBD-rich products for dogs; its naturally low THC (below 0.3%) eliminates the potential for psychoactivity or toxicity in dogs.

Since the 1960s, scientists have demonstrated dozens of therapeutic applications for CBD and other non-psychoactive cannabinoids (and terpenes, another class of chemical compounds) present in hemp, which we will explore in the coming chapters of this book.

The last few years have been revolutionary in the recognition of CBD as a therapeutic agent. The turning point for the public was in 2013, when neurosurgeon Dr. Sanjay Gupta researched the topic and presented his findings in a series of media reports for CNN, concluding:

"I apologize because I didn't look hard enough, until now. I didn't look far enough… We have been terribly and systematically misled for nearly 70 years in the United States, and I apologize for my own role in that."[2]

Initially a skeptic, Gupta became a major proponent for the use of medical marijuana, and particularly advocated the heightened beneficial use of CBD in association with other cannabinoids, the so-called entourage effect.[3]

For the purposes of this book, the primary benefits of industrial hemp are found in CBD and other non-psychoactive cannabinoids and terpenes, with CBD being the book's primary focus.

MARIJUANA VERSUS HEMP PRODUCTS FOR PETS

Narda Robinson, DO, DVM, of Colorado State University, is the preeminent veterinary authority on the use of cannabis for pets. Dr. Robinson shares the following in her article "The Latest on Cannabis and Hemp for Pets," *Veterinary Practice News,* September 2015.[4]

> Because marijuana falls under the Schedule I classification, it is illegal for veterinarians to prescribe. Drug Enforcement Administration officials are quick to remind practitioners that their DEA license is based on federal, not state, laws.[i]
>
> The Veterinary Medical Examining Board of Oregon states plainly on its website that "Marijuana is not approved for veterinary use" and that a veterinarian may not write a prescription for "pet marijuana."[ii]

The AVMA news site states that it is illegal for veterinarians to recommend medical marijuana.

In contrast, a legislator from Nevada has introduced a bill proposing "pet medical marijuana cards" for veterinary conditions that might be helped by marijuana.[iii]

However, veterinarians cannot determine which medical problems marijuana might help without research, and Schedule I restrictions on marijuana research impose high barriers to further study.

i. Personal communication with a DEA representative at the AVMA Convention in Boston. July 2015.

ii. Veterinary Medical Examining Board. Oregon.gov. Accessed at http://www.oregon.gov/ovmeb/Pages/index.aspx on 07-27-15.

iii. Glionna, JM. Medical marijuana for dogs and cats? Nevada lawmaker says yes. *Los Angeles Times.* March 18, 2015. Accessed at http://www.latimes.com/nation/la-na-pet-pot-20150317-story.html on 07-27-15.

Current laws on both the federal and local level, as well as DEA regulations for veterinary medical professionals nationwide, make it impossible at this time to recommend any marijuana-based products for pets, period.

Industrial hemp products, on the other hand, suffer from none of these limitations.

IN REVIEW:

- Cannabis has been used for medicinal purposes since ancient times and was widely marketed by major pharmaceuticals until the 1937 Marihuana Act.
- Although marijuana and industrial hemp belong to the same species, marijuana is the cultivar with high THC used for psychoactive and recreational purposes, and industrial hemp is the cultivar with low THC used for fiber, food and non-psychoactive purposes.
- Hemp is an organic, non-GMO crop, legally grown in 98% of the world, and has been in the animal food supply for millennia.
- On average, hemp has a vastly higher level of CBD compared to marijuana; CBD is at least as (and potentially much more) important than THC when it comes to the therapeutic potential for medicinal cannabis.
- It is illegal for veterinarians to prescribe marijuana products, but legal for anyone to buy and use hemp products without any prescriptions at all.

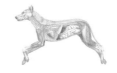

CHAPTER 2:

CANNABIS, CANNABINOIDS, AND THE ENDOCANNABINOID SYSTEM

n 2900 BCE, Chinese Emperor Fu Hsi noted that cannabis was a very popular medicine that possessed both yin and yang.

In 1500 BCE it was included in the Chinese pharmacopeia, the Rh-Ya.

The book of Exodus talks of holy anointing oil from cannabis. "The sacred character of hemp in biblical times is evident from Exodus 30:23, where Moses was instructed by God to anoint the meeting tent and all of its furnishings with specially prepared oil, containing hemp."[1]

Exodus   כִּי תִשָּׂא

רֹאשׁ מָר־דְּרוֹר חֲמֵשׁ מֵאוֹת וְקִנְּמָן־בֶּשֶׂם מַחֲצִיתוֹ חֲמִשִּׁים
וּמָאתַיִם (וּקְנֵה־בֹשֶׂם) חֲמִשִּׁים וּמָאתָיִם : וְקִדָּה חֲמֵשׁ   24
מֵאוֹת בְּשֶׁקֶל הַקֹּדֶשׁ וְשֶׁמֶן זַיִת הִין : וְעָשִׂיתָ אֹתוֹ שֶׁמֶן   25
מִשְׁחַת־קֹדֶשׁ רֹקַח מִרְקַחַת מַעֲשֵׂה רֹקֵחַ שֶׁמֶן מִשְׁחַת־
קֹדֶשׁ יִהְיֶה : וּמָשַׁחְתָּ בוֹ אֶת־אֹהֶל מוֹעֵד וְאֵת אֲרוֹן הָעֵדֻת :   26
וְאֶת־הַשֻּׁלְחָן וְאֶת־כָּל־כֵּלָיו וְאֶת־הַמְּנֹרָה וְאֶת־כֵּלֶיהָ וְאֵת   27
מִזְבַּח הַקְּטֹרֶת : וְאֶת־מִזְבַּח הָעֹלָה וְאֶת־כָּל־כֵּלָיו וְאֶת־   28
הַכִּיֹּר וְאֶת־כַּנּוֹ : וְקִדַּשְׁתָּ אֹתָם וְהָיוּ קֹדֶשׁ קָדָשִׁים כָּל־   29
הַנֹּגֵעַ בָּהֶם יִקְדָּשׁ :

— fragrant cane. *Keneh bosem* in Hebrew. Ancient sources identify this with the sweet calamus (Septuagint; Rambam on Kerithoth 1:1; Saadia; Ibn Janach). This is the sweetflag or flag-root, *Acoras calamus* which grows in Europe. It appears that a similar species grew in the Holy Land, in the Hula region in ancient times (Theophrastus, *History of Plants* 9:7). Other sources apparently indicate that it was the Indian plant, *Cympo-pogan martini*, which has the form of red straw (*Yad, Kley HaMikdash* 1:3).

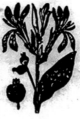
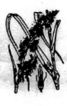
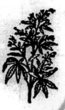

Canna   Cympopogan   Hemp

On the basis of cognate pronunciation and Septuagint readings, some identify *Keneh bosem* with the English and Greek cannabis, the hemp plant.

There are, however, some authorities who identify the "sweet cane" with cinnamon bark (Radak, *Sherashim*). Some say that *kinman* is the wood, and *keneh bosem* is the bark (Abarbanel).

30:24 cassia (Radak, *Sherashim*; *Peshita*; Vulgate). *Kidah* in Hebrew; *ketzia* in Aramaic (*Targum*; Rambam on *Kelayim* 1:8). Cassia is the common name for the bark of the tree *Cin-namomum cassia* or *Cassia lignea* belonging to the laurel family, which grows in China. (*Pachad Yitzchak*, s.v. *Ketoreth*; cf. Pliny 12:43; Theophrastus, *History of Plants* 9:7; Diodorus Siculus 3:46; Herodatus 3:110).

There are some, however, who identify the "cassia" of the ancients, and hence *kidah* here, with costus, known as *kosht* in the Talmud (*Yad, Kley HaMikdash* 1:3; Saadia; Ibn Janach; cf. Rashi). Costus is the root of the annual herb, *Saussurea lappa*, which grows on the mountain slopes of Kashmir, and is used for incense and perfume.

Cassia

The Septuagint translates *kidah* here as *iris*, possibly *Castus speciosus*. Others suggest that it is kitto or mosylon, a plant very much like cassia, coming from Meuzel on the African coast (cf. Dioscorides, *De Materia Medica* 1:13).

— gallon. *Hin* in Hebrew. Actually 0.97 gallon, or 3.6 liter.

30:25 blended compound. The anointing oil was made by soaking the aromatic substances in water until the essential essences are extracted. The oil is then placed over the water, and the water slowly cooked away, allowing the essences to mix with the oil (*Yad, Kley HaMikdash* 1:2; from *Kerithoth* 5a). According to another opinion, the oil was cooked with the aromatic herbs, and then filtered out (*Ibid.*).

The ancient Egyptians used cannabis and cannabis oil for glaucoma, inflammation and enemas, referencing them in The Ebers Papyrus (c. 1550 BCE) which is the one of the first medical textbooks in recorded history.

The ancient Greeks used cannabis to dress wounds and sores on their horses. In humans, dried leaves of cannabis were used to treat nosebleeds, and cannabis seeds were used to expel tapeworms. The most frequently described use of cannabis in humans was to steep green seeds of cannabis in either water or wine, remove the seeds, and use the warm extract to treat inflammation and pain resulting from obstruction of the ear.[2]

Indian medicine expanded the medicinal uses of cannabis, using all parts of the plant for some sort of illness or another (whether physical or spiritual) and led the charge in holistic and herbal medicine. Specifically, the Atharvaveda (1000 BCE) makes reference to medicinal cannabis, which is described as one of five sacred

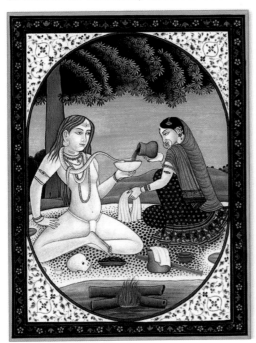

plants within the five kingdoms of herbs that release us from anxiety.

Cannabis, medicinally speaking, was recommended in India to quicken the mind, give strength and agility, achieve spiritual freedom and higher consciousness, lower fevers, stimulate appetite, improve digestion and relieve headaches.

A mixture of cannabis and milk was used as an anesthetic in India.[3]

And so it goes around the world, through history: cannabis is used to treat leprosy, earaches, edema, gout, joint cramps, pain, migraines, vomiting, hemorrhage, diarrhea, anorexia, depression, arthritis, menstrual cramps, headaches, insomnia, neuralgia, convulsions, opium addiction—and on and on. How could one plant treat so many diverse ailments?

It took thousands of years before the answer revealed itself, and in so doing, it opened the door to one of the most exciting and revolutionary medical advancements of our time. It turns out that medical cannabis doesn't work by getting you high. Instead, it works by way of a hitherto unknown system in the body that affects how almost every other system works: the endocannabinoid system (ECS), named after the cannabis plant.

THE ENDOCANNABINOID SYSTEM

The endocannabinoid system consists of a group of specialized receptors in the brain and peripheral nervous system of all vertebrates. It is involved in a variety of physiological processes including appetite, pain sensation, nausea, or mood, memory, and inflammation.[4]

In 1964, Dr. Ralph Mechoulam identified tetrahydrocannabinol (THC) as the chemical in marijuana responsible for making people feel high. But that didn't fully explain how cannabis quelled nausea or seizures, dampened nausea, or lessened pain. Experiments showed it didn't work with the endorphin system or any other known system. Where were cannabinoid receptor sites in the brain?

It turns out, just about everywhere. In the late 1980s, scientists found receptor sites all over the brain that reacted to THC. These

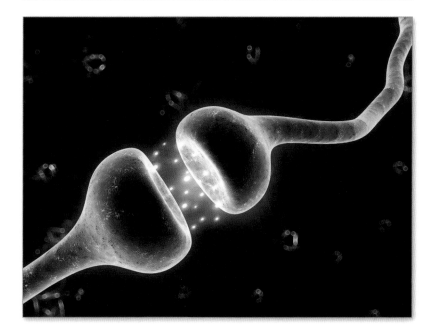

cannabinoid receptors, CB1 as they called them, were more abundant in the brain than any other kind of neurotransmitter receptor.

Then scientists discovered a second type of cannabinoid receptor, which they called CB2 as opposed to the first type, CB1. While CB1 receptors are mostly in the brain and central nervous system, CB2 receptors are mostly in the peripheral cells, especially immune system cells. To a lesser extent, CB1 receptors are also in the lungs, blood vessels, muscles, digestive tract, and reproductive organs. CB2 receptors are also in the liver, bone marrow, pancreas, and brainstem. In other words, they're all over!

Here's how they work: The cells in your (and your pet's) brain and nervous system communicate with each other by means of various types of chemicals called neurotransmitters. Specific chemicals are released from the end of one nerve cell, travel across a tiny gap, and fit into a receptor site on the beginning of the next nerve cell.

Once the next nerve cell is activated, that cell releases its own endogenous cannabinoids, which travel backward across the same gap to the nerve cell that released the neurotransmitter, attach to a cannabinoid receptor on that nerve cell, and tell the nerve cell to cut down on releasing the neurotransmitter. It acts sort of like a thermostat.

The body produces its own neurotransmitters (called endogenous neurotransmitters) and its own endogenous cannabinoids. Each of the types of neurotransmitters and cannabinoids fit only in certain receptors because the receptor is shaped so it only accepts certain shaped chemicals, like a lock and key.

Many drugs work because they have the exact or nearly exact shape as a particular endogenous neurotransmitter. For example, the active chemical in opium is morphine, which has a chemical shape similar to endorphins, a type of feel-good chemical the brain makes when the body feels pain. Morphine locks into those same endorphin receptor sites and alleviates pain.

But why would our bodies have receptors for a plant chemical? It turns out that just as we naturally produce our own endorphins, we also naturally produce our own endogenous cannabinoids: endocannabinoids or what some have dubbed our "inner cannabis." Scientists named the first endocannabinoid they discovered "anandamine," from the Sanskrit word "ananda," meaning bliss. The plant chemicals (phytochemicals) found in cannabis closely mimic the body's endogenous cannabinoids. Thus, when cannabinoids from cannabis interact with cannabinoid receptors, they elicit the same response as would the body's endogenous cannabinoids. No wonder cannabis can impact so many body systems!

The endocannabinoid system isn't something just humans—or even mammals—can lay claim to. It's evolutionarily ancient, found in primitive animals 600 million years ago, and all mammals, birds, reptiles, and fish today—in fact, pretty much every animal but insects.[5] In 2005 it was hypothesized that the evolution of cannabinoid receptors was linked to the evolution of multi-cellular animals.[6] Scientists suspected that to be so ubiquitous, endocannabinoids and the endocannabinoid system must be doing something very important.

They are. Endocannabinoids modulate *every other neurotransmitter*. They're like the master regulator, telling some to speed it up and others to calm it down, directing some to fight problems and others to restore the body to its normal state. When we have

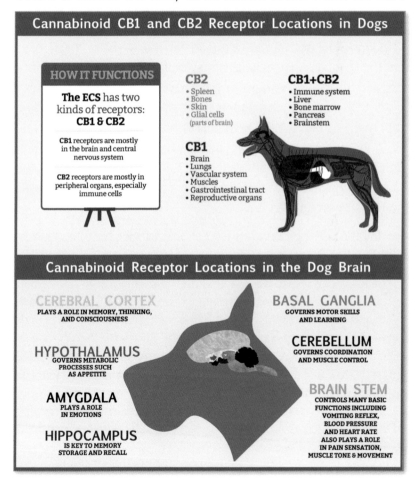

an infection, endocannabinoid signals tell the immune system to turn up the temperature to fight it, and when the invader is destroyed, they signal it to turn it back down. And endocannabinoids do this sort of thing in system after system, balancing all the other systems to maintain the body's homeostasis.

The common misconception for many years was that THC was the only cannabinoid responsible for influencing health. It is not. Far from it.

BEYOND THC: CANNABIDIOL AND OTHER CANNABINOIDS

THC is just one of many cannabinoids present in cannabis. Although THC got all the attention for many years, these days another cannabinoid, called cannabidiol (CBD), is the one that's causing all the excitement in the medical community. Not only does CBD lack the psychoactive effects of THC, but it appears that many of the health benefits THC has been getting the credit for in therapeutic cannabis are actually the work of CBD and other non-psychoactive cannabinoids. CBD doesn't get you high, and non-psychoactive cannabinoids have much higher safety levels and toxicity limits than THC.

In fact, the U.S. government filed U.S. Patent 6630507 for cannabidiol way back in 1999, stating:

> Cannabinoids have been found to have antioxidant properties, unrelated to NMDA receptor antagonism. This new found property makes cannabinoids useful in the treatment and prophylaxis of wide variety of oxidation associated diseases, such as ischemic, age-related, inflammatory and autoimmune diseases. The cannabinoids are found to have particular application as neuroprotectants, for example in limiting neurological damage following ischemic insults, such as stroke and trauma, or in the treatment of neurodegenerative diseases, such as Alzheimer's disease, Parkinson's disease and HIV dementia. Nonpsychoactive cannabinoids, such as cannabidiol, are particularly advantageous to use because they avoid toxicity that is

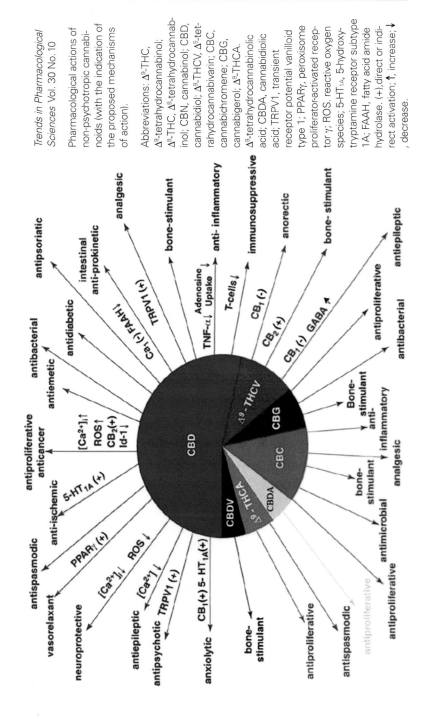

Trends in Pharmacological Sciences Vol. 30 No. 10

Pharmacological actions of non-psychotropic cannabinoids (with the indication of the proposed mechanisms of action).

Abbreviations: Δ⁹-THC, Δ⁹-tetrahydrocannabinol; Δ⁸-THC, Δ⁸-tetrahydrocannabinol; CBN, cannabinol; CBD, cannabidiol; Δ⁹-THCV, Δ⁹-tetrahydrocannabivarin; CBC, cannabichromene; CBG, cannabigerol; Δ⁹-THCA, Δ⁹-tetrahydrocannabinolic acid; CBDA, cannabidiolic acid; TRPV1, transient receptor potential vanilloid type 1; PPARγ, peroxisome proliferator-activated receptor γ; ROS, reactive oxygen species; 5-HT₁ₐ, 5-hydroxytryptamine receptor subtype 1A; FAAH, fatty acid amide hydrolase. (+),direct or indirect activation; ↑, increase; ↓, decrease.

encountered with psychoactive cannabinoids at high doses useful in the method of the present invention.[7]

A 2009 article reviewing the therapeutic actions of non-psychoactive cannabinoids found 76 reports on their efficacy—and more than half of the therapeutic effects were attributed to CBD. These included anti-anxiety, antipsychotic, antiepileptic, neuroprotective, blood vessel relaxant, antispasmodic, anticancer, antinausea, antidiabetic, analgesic, antibacterial, anti-inflammatory, immunosuppressive, bone stimulant, and more!

Beyond CBD there are many other non-psychoactive cannabinoids with potential health benefits. ß-caryophyllene (BCP), cannabidivarin (CBDV), cannabigerol (CBG), cannabichromene (CBC), and cannabidiolic acid (CBDA) have all demonstrated effects.

PHYTOCANNABINOIDS

Phytocannabinoids are cannabinoids produced by plants. The cannabis plant expresses an abundant amount of cannabinoids, and breeding has determined whether those are skewed toward THC

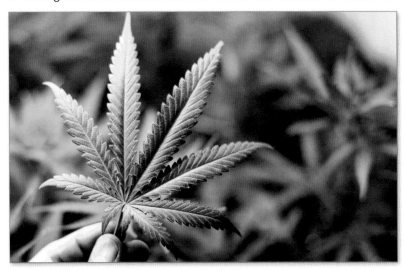

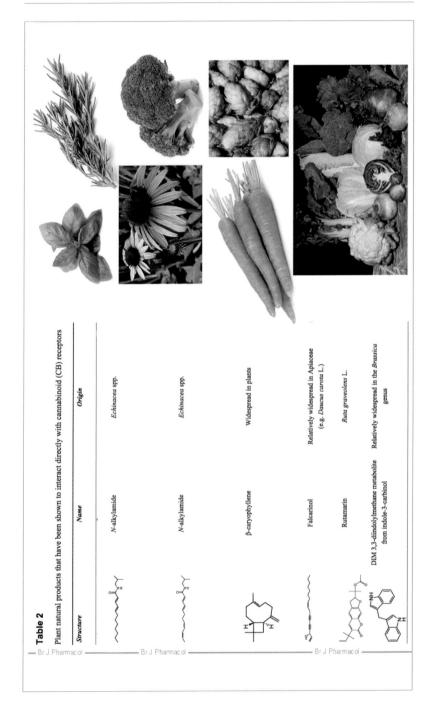

Table 2

Plant natural products that have been shown to interact directly with cannabinoid (CB) receptors

Structure	Name	Origin
	N-alkylamide	Echinacea spp.
	N-alkylamide	Echinacea spp.
	β-caryophyllene	Widespread in plants
	Falcarinol	Relatively widespread in Apiaceae (e.g. Daucus carota L.)
	Rutamarin	Ruta graveolens L.
	DIM 3,3-diindolylmethane metabolite from indole-3-carbinol	Relatively widespread in the Brassica genus

(as in marijuana) or toward the non-psychoactive cannabinoids (as in industrial hemp and ancient medicinal cannabis).

Decades of breeding for psychoactive THC content has resulted in the majority of marijuana forms of the plant being nearly devoid of other cannabinoids.

On the other hand, industrial hemp plants do not express significant THC, and instead turn their cannabinoid production to CBD. Industrial hemp plants also contain CBG, CBC, and many other beneficial cannabinoids, some or all of which may have a synergistic effect on one another.

For example, the cannabinoid ß-caryophyllene (BCP) is present in hemp and increases the body's uptake of CBD. Traditionally labeled a terpene, it was only recently discovered to be a cannabinoid that binds the CB2 receptor.[8] BCP is actually present in many other plants such as rosemary, basil, and especially black pepper. ß-caryophyllene was the first "dietary cannabinoid"— that is, a cannabinoid widespread in the traditional food system, and *already an FDA-approved food additive.* And it, too, acts as a powerful anti-inflammatory.[9]

Although cannabis has the highest levels and variety of cannabinoids, phytocannabinoids can also be found in some other plants, such as broccoli, carrots, cauliflower, echinacea, flax, green tea, oregano, and many other vegetables widely accepted to be healthy. They've been part of our diet for centuries, but most cannabinoids are not present in other plants to the extent they are in cannabis. Cannabis, specifically the industrial hemp form, is the most abundant plant source of CBD in the world.

IN REVIEW:

- Cannabis has a 5,000-year history as a food and therapeutic product.
- The body's neural cells communicate by means of endogenous chemicals that fit in receptors in a lock and key manner; other chemicals of similar shape can sometimes fit into the same receptors and cause the same reaction.
- Cannabinoids found in many plants fit into the body's cannabinoid receptor sites, which regulate other neurotransmitters as well as a host of body systems, especially the immune system.
- Cannabidiol (CBD) is a non-psychoactive cannabinoid found in greatest abundance in industrial hemp; CBD is emerging as the most important cannabinoid for health.

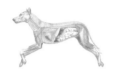

CHAPTER 3:

CLINICAL APPLICATIONS FOR CANNABINOIDS

Although cannabis has been used medicinally for centuries, only recently have scientific studies documented its effectiveness. That research is ongoing, but at present there are more than 13,000 journal articles on cannabinoids and more than 1500 on cannabidiol[1] (CBD) specifically.[2] Cannabinoids show promise in a vast array of applications, many of which have been studied in animal models over the past three decades.

Evidence for cannabinoids' efficacy comes from several sources. First, peer-reviewed journal articles. These are the gold standard of scientific evidence, as any report is rigorously reviewed, questioned, and critiqued by fellow scientists before it's allowed to be published. Second, scientific studies conducted for private companies. These may undergo the same rigorous scrutiny but may not be published in regular journals. Finally, anecdotal reports, while not subject to scrutiny, may be suggestive of results.

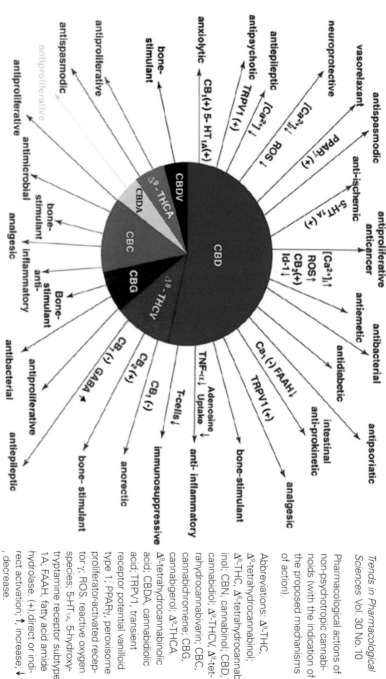

Pharmacological actions of non-psychotropic cannabinoids (with the indication of the proposed mechanisms of action).

Abbreviations: Δ⁹-THC, Δ⁹-tetrahydrocannabinol; Δ⁸-THC, Δ⁸-tetrahydrocannabinol; CBN, cannabinol; CBD, cannabidiol; Δ⁹-THCV, Δ⁹-tetrahydrocannabivarin; CBC, cannabichromene; CBG, cannabigerol; Δ⁹-THCA, Δ⁹-tetrahydrocannabinolic acid; CBDA, cannabidiolic acid; TRPV1, transient receptor potential vanilloid type 1; PPARγ, peroxisome proliferator-activated receptor γ; ROS, reactive oxygen species; 5-HT₁ₐ, 5-hydroxytryptamine receptor subtype 1A; FAAH, fatty acid amide hydrolase. (+),direct or indirect activation; ↑, increase; ↓, decrease.

The peer-reviewed journal *Trends in Pharmacological Sciences* printed a survey article in 2009 that summarized 76 published scientific reports from 1980-2009 to generate the above chart of pharmacological actions of non-psychotropic cannabinoids.[3] The diverse and tremendous potential for these phytochemicals is apparent.

In the past ten years many clinical applications have come to light as cannabinoid research has dramatically expanded in the U.S. and globally. A few of them are highlighted in this chapter.

"FIRST, DO NO HARM."

An extensive review in 2011 looked for any evidence that CBD could have harmful effects. CBD was found to be non-toxic, with very few, if any, side effects.[4]

CBD can theoretically inhibit metabolism of drugs that rely on the liver (specifically cytochrome P450s 3A, 2C and 2B subfamilies) to metabolize them; it is probably wise to err on the side of caution and discontinue CBD for a few days before giving such drugs, which can include some dewormers and heartworm preventives. Owners should consult with their veterinarian before combining such drugs with CBD.

Much research has been conducted on the potential addictive properties of cannabis. Marijuana—the kind with high levels of THC—is in fact mildly addictive. Hemp, with low THC and high CBD, is not. CBD lacks the hedonic attributes of THC and is neither mentally nor physically addictive. In fact, study after study has shown that CBD actually has anti-addictive properties, and is actually beneficial in treating addictions to alcohol, tobacco, opiates, marijuana, and psychostimulants in people and animals.[5]

The list of conditions CBD seems to help is exploding. The discovery of the cannabinoid receptor system has opened up an entirely new world for research and potential health benefits. Much more research needs to be done, but the following, all from peer-reviewed journal articles, are just some examples of what researchers have already found.

ANXIETY

Anxiety in people and pets can be disruptive, even debilitating. Separation anxiety, noise phobias triggered by thunder or fireworks, and fear of strange people, animals, or situations are all too common in pets. Areas of the brain (such as the prefrontal cortex, amygdala, and hippocampus) involved in mood, stress, and fear are rich in cannabinoid receptors. CB1 receptors are known to be involved in mediating fearfulness and anxiety. Mice bred without CB1 receptors, or mice in which other drugs block the CB1 receptors, are constantly fearful and anxious. In contrast, cannabinoids boost CB1 receptors and produce a calming, or anxiolytic, effect.

CBD is known to help treat many human mental health problems, including anxiety. In a 2012 review of studies examining CBD's effect on anxiety, the authors noted that "recent studies have shown that CBD exerts inherent anxiolytic effects, both in rodent models [157,198-201] and, more recently, in patients affected by social phobia [202,203]... CBD has been shown to reduce amygdalar responses to fearful stimuli [207]; this mechanism may be essential for the anxiolytic effects of this compound in social phobia [203]. Furthermore, CBD has been shown to elicit antipanic effects through the activation of 5-HT1A receptors in the dorsal periaqueductal gray, a critical area for the modulation of emotional reactivity to stress [208,209]."[6]

A 2014 review concluded that "the anxiolytic and antipsychotic properties of CBD stand out. CBD's anxiolytic effects are apparently similar to those of approved drugs to treat anxiety."[7]

AGING AND MENTAL FUNCTION

Pets and people can suffer from loss of mental abilities with age. Cognitive Dysfunction Syndrome is considered the animal correlate to human Alzheimer's disease. People with Alzheimer's exhibit dramatically reduced functioning of cannabinoid receptors in the brain. They also have increased plaque deposits along with microglia, which cause inflammation.

Multiple cannabinoids exhibit neuroprotective, anti-inflammatory and antioxidant properties that may be important in protecting nerve cells. When rats injected with substances that correlate with plaque formation are also given cannabinoids, they perform better in tests of mental ability than those not receiving cannabinoids. Analyses of their brains show that cannabinoids prevent activation of microglia and thus have reduced inflammation—all leading to preservation of mental function![8]

Now researchers have found CBD helps regenerate new neurons in the part of the brain (the hippocampus) responsible for memory. And when CBD is administered to animals with memory loss, their memory improves![9]

ARTHRITIS

Pets suffer from both osteoarthritis (the kind associated with age) and rheumatoid arthritis (the kind associated with autoimmune disease). CBD reduces inflammation and pain, decreasing the symptoms of both types of arthritis. CBD blocks disease progression in a mouse model of rheumatoid arthritis, both protecting the joints against severe damage and inhibiting the release of tumor necrosis factor that causes joint inflammation and destruction. CBD acts as both an immunosuppressant and anti-inflammatory to achieve these results.[10] Other cannabinoids that act as anti-inflammatories are CBG, CBC, CBGA, CBCA, THCA, CBDA, and BCP.

AUTOIMMUNE DISORDERS

Dogs are prone to several autoimmune disorders, notably auto-immune thyroiditis, immune-mediated hemolytic anemia and/or thrombocytopenia, pemphigus, lupus, some arthritis and pos-sibly sudden acquired retinal degeneration syndrome, among others. In autoimmune disorders, the body's immune system attacks normal cells in the body as though they were invaders. It may target cells in the thyroid, blood, joints, eye, skin, and even some internal organs. Cannabinoids affect almost every compo-nent of the immune system,[11] leading researchers to investigate their effect in preventing autoimmune disease. It's believed that inflammation may set off an immune response, which then either misidentifies the target or fails to turn off. Because cannabinoids decrease inflammation, they may be the first step in preventing autoimmune disease. Other mechanisms may also be at play. For example, cannabinoids alter microRNAs, which are known to act as brakes on the immune system.[12]

BONE HEALTH

Like people, pets can suffer from bone loss, or osteoporosis, with age, and broken bones are all too common. CBD both prevents osteoporosis and helps heal fractures. Cannabinoid receptors as well as endogenous cannabinoids are found throughout the skel-etal system. The CB2 receptor stimulates bone formation and inhibits bone loss.[13] CBD has been shown to prevent bone loss in aged rodents and to promote healing after fractures. In fact, the bones in treated animals were 35–50% stronger than those in untreated ones![14] CBD, CBG, CBC and THCV are all cannabinoids that have been found to be bone stimulants.

CANCER

Long-standing inflammation predisposes to cancer, possibly due to the free radicals and oxidative damage. For whatever reason, inflammation encourages the survival of cells with mutations that allow them to grow unchecked. Most cells naturally grow old and die, a process called apoptosis. But these cancer cells never die. They encourage new blood vessels to grow to support them, edge out normal cells, overflow their bounds, and grow into tumors, or just start taking over the bloodstream. In addition, malignant cancer cells are better than normal cells at moving from one place in the body to another.

An extensive review by the National Cancer Institute documented mounting evidence that cannabinoids not only help manage symptoms of cancer and its treatment, such as pain, nausea, and fatigue, but more importantly, reduce inflammation, induce cancer cells to die, slow cancer growth, inhibit the formation of blood vessels that feed tumors, and protect non-cancer cells.[15]

As early as 1998, cannabinoids were shown to induce cell death in glioma cells that make up a very aggressive form of brain cancer. Since then, study after study has shown that cannabinoids inhibit cancer cell growth, induce cancer cells to die, and inhibit cancer cell invasion and metastasis[16]—and unlike traditional chemotherapies, they do this without hurting normal cells. In fact, they may even protect them.

These results have been demonstrated in peer-reviewed studies of brain cancer, breast cancer, colon cancer, lung cancer, prostate cancer, bladder cancer, melanoma, and leukemia, and the evidence comes from petri-dish cell lines, animal models, and even clinical trials. What's more, CBD given along with chemotherapy seems to increase the effectiveness of the chemotherapy drugs. Cannabinoids aren't just for treating cancer; there's also evidence they may reduce the risk of developing cancer because of their anti-inflammatory effects. According to a 2005 report in *Mini-Reviews in Medicinal Chemistry*, cannabinoids "may represent a new class of anticancer drugs that retard cancer growth, inhibit angiogenesis and the metastatic spreading of cancer cells."[17] Other cannabinoids with anti-proliferative properties include CBG, CBC, THCA, and CBDA.

COLITIS

People and pets can both suffer from gastrointestinal disorders, with inflammatory bowel disease (IBD) particularly common and resistant to therapy. Studies have now shown that cannabis is helpful in many gastrointestinal diseases, including IBD. Cannabinoids reduce gastrointestinal mobility and inflammation, and have been heralded as a new therapeutic strategy to treat IBD.[18] CBD-rich industrial hemp has been shown to decrease intestinal motility more than THC-rich Indian hemp.[19]

DEGENERATIVE MYELOPATHY

The effect of cannabis on amyotrophic lateral sclerosis (ALS), better known as Lou Gehrig's disease, is of interest to dog owners because of the widespread occurrence of its canine counterpart, degenerative myelopathy (DM). Because of the similarities of the disease, cannabis may offer new hope in preventing or treating DM in pets. When mice bred to develop ALS were given cannabis, their disease was delayed; when it did appear, it progressed more slowly than those not given cannabis. The researchers concluded that "Based on the currently available scientific data, it is reasonable to think that cannabis might significantly slow the progression of ALS, potentially extending life expectancy and substantially reducing the overall burden of the disease."[20] As DNA testing can identify many at-risk dogs, it seems reasonable to try to slow or prevent the disease progression with cannabis.

DIABETES

Dogs and cats are both susceptible to diabetes. The condition is difficult to control, and many people cannot cope with the demands of treating a diabetic pet. Cannabinoids may offer help. With cannabinoids' role as master controller of hormones and other neurotransmitters involved in homeostasis, it's no surprise that they influence metabolism. Interestingly, human cannabis users are more likely to possess a lower body mass index, lower fasting insulin, and lower insulin resistance compared to non-users.[21]

Chronic inflammation plays a key role in the development of type 2 diabetes. CBD's anti-inflammatory properties may lessen inflammation and reduce the chance of developing diabetes. CBD has been shown to reduce the incidence of diabetes in normal-weight mice,[22] and it may actually suppress and even reverse the disease.[23]

A second cannabinoid, THCV (tetrahydrocannabivarin), has also been shown to combat diabetes. A 2013 study reported that THCV reduces glucose intolerance, improves glucose tolerance, improves liver triglyceride levels, and increases insulin sensitivity—all beneficial relative to diabetes.[24]

FREE RADICALS

Most people know free radicals are bad, but few understand why. Free radicals are involved in aging, cancer, and other significant diseases. They occur when cell molecules have an unpaired electron, causing them to be unstable and to capture an additional electron from adjacent stable molecules. If they succeed, those molecules in turn become free radicals, and the process continues until they disrupt the cell they make up.

Aging, along with environmental factors such as pollution, radiation, herbicides, and cigarette smoke, increase free radical damage. The body normally produces antioxidants that neutralize free radicals, but if free radicals become too abundant, cell damage can occur.

CBD acts as an antioxidant, and may be helpful in preventing or treating a number of conditions brought on or worsened by free radicals. In fact, the United States government holds a patent for using cannabinoids as antioxidants and neuroprotectants.[25]

GLAUCOMA

Pets, especially dogs, can suffer from glaucoma, a state of increased pressure within the eye that can cause pain and blindness. Cannabis has long been known to alleviate glaucoma to some degree, but THC has been the component most associated with this relief. A recent study using cats found another cannabinoid, cannabigerol (CBG), is equally effective and doesn't have THC's mind-altering properties.[26]

INFECTIONS

All the major cannabinoids, including CBD, have been shown to have potent action against many bacteria, most notably methicillin-resistant Staphylococcus aureus (MRSA).[27]) MRSA occurs in pets just as it does in people. CBD also has antibacterial power against staphylococci and streptococci.[28] CBG has antibacterial properties (Mechoulam and Gaoni 1965), and so does CBCA.[29]

INFLAMMATION

Dogs and other pets can suffer from a variety of inflammatory diseases, including arthritis, asthma, inflammatory bowel disease, conjunctivitis, dermatitis, glomerulonephritis, masticatory muscle myositis, pancreatitis, panosteitis, and uveitis—basically any disease ending in "itis."

Many human physicians and researchers now believe the role of inflammation in the creation and proliferation of disease is far greater than previously thought. "Inflammation is the root of cancer, heart disease and brain decline," says David Agus, M.D., Professor of Medicine and Engineering at the University of Southern California and author of *The End of Illness: A Short Guide to a Long Life*.

Tanya Edwards, M.D., the founder and former Medical Director of Cleveland Clinic's Center for Integrative Medicine, writes that inflammation is now recognized as the underlying basis of a significant number of diseases. Research has shown that inflammation plays a role in turning on genes that predispose an animal to certain diseases, including cancer. Edwards writes that Alzheimer's disease, cardiovascular disease, and diabetes, among others, may all be related to chronic inflammation in the human body.[30]

CB2 receptors appear to be critical targets for regulating inflammation, and cannabinoids have been shown to be effective in suppressing inflammation all over the body. Cannabinoids suppress inflammatory responses, and thus lessen disease symptoms. They protect against autoimmune disorders. And they may be helpful in preventing certain types of cancers triggered by chronic inflammation. Cannabinoids with documented anti-inflammatory properties include cannabidiol (CBD), ß-caryophyllene (BCP), cannabigerol (CBG), cannabichromene (CBC), cannabigerolic acid (CBGa), and cannabidiolic acid (CBDa).

A 2009 review of cannabinoids concluded, "[c]annabinoids are potent anti-inflammatory agents" and that "[m]anipulation of endocannabinoids and/or use of exogenous cannabinoids *in vivo* can constitute a potent treatment modality against inflammatory disorders."[31]

OBESITY

Obesity is at epidemic proportions among pets and people. Although THC is well-known for increasing appetite, surprisingly, people who use cannabis are documented to have lower prevalence of obesity, with lower body mass index and smaller waist size compared to non-users[32] despite the fact that they consume more calories.[33] The effect is postulated to be due to the combined actions of several cannabinoids, especially CBD and THCV. There are anecdotal reports of people taking CBD who had reduced appetite and weight loss, but the question awaits more rigorous research.

OBSESSIVE-COMPULSIVE DISORDER (OCD)

OCD occurs in animals as well as people; in fact, a genetic basis for it has been found in some dog breeds. The condition in animals can be debilitating, as it may involve self-mutilation or chronic repetitive behavior at the cost of interacting with family or even eating.

Anecdotal reports from people with OCD support the finding that CBD reduces obsessive-compulsive behaviors. Even at low doses, CBD has been shown to decrease repetitive behavior in rats.[34]

PAIN

Cannabinoids achieve anlagesia, or pain reduction, through CBD1 receptors in parts of the brain responsible for pain reception (nociception) and CBD2 receptors in peripheral nerve endings. Cannabinoids also alleviate pain by causing other cells to reduce their release of inflammatory agents. Cannabinoids prevent neuropathy in animals exposed to chemotherapy drugs[35] and can be as effective as morphine in the reduction of tumor pain.[36]

Numerous cannabinoids, including CBD, CBG, CBN, CBCA, and CBGA have demonstrated analgesic properties.

Bone cancer is a particularly painful tumor seen in pets. Several studies have shown cannabinoids can reduce this pain.[37]

SEIZURES

Medical marijuana is probably best known for its ability to quell intractable seizures, and in fact it has been used for this for centuries. Decades of research have shown that cannabinoids, including CBD and cannabidivaran (CBDV) effectively control seizures in animal models.[38] CBD affects several endogenous cannabinoid pathways simultaneously and works additively and sometimes synergistically with other anti-epileptic drugs.[39]

The widely publicized case of a young girl named Charlotte, who had intractable seizures, brought the use of medical marijuana to the public's attention.[40] Most people don't realize it was CBD-rich extract, rather than THC, that brought about her dramatic reduction in seizure rate from about 1,200 a month to about three. She's not alone. Of nearly 40 epileptic children, all but one saw such vast improvement that they were removed from their regular medication.

Seizures also occur in pets, especially some dog breeds, and many result in euthanasia. Anecdotal reports and user surveys confirm that cannabinoids can dramatically reduce seizure rates and intensity in dogs, but no published studies are yet available.

SKIN CONDITIONS

The most common skin condition of pets is pruritis (itchiness). The condition can be so bad that pet owners turn to euthanasia.

Now CBD may offer an option. Sensory nerve fibers from the skin contain cannabinoid receptors. Researchers found that cannabinoids applied directly to the skin can significantly reduce itching in humans.[41] Other studies have also found that cannabinoids can protect against contact dermatitis.[42]

A review article about the role of cannabinoids in skin health concludes: "It seems that the main physiological function of the cutaneous ECS is to constitutively control the proper and well-balanced proliferation, differentiation and survival, as well as immune competence and/or tolerance, of skin cells. The disruption of this delicate balance might facilitate the development of multiple pathological conditions and diseases of the skin (e.g., acne, seborrhea, allergic dermatitis, itch and pain, psoriasis, hair growth disorders, systemic sclerosis and cancer)."[43]

Another, which looked specifically at cannabinoid receptors in dog skin, concluded: "The endocannabinoid system and cannabimimetic compounds protect against effects of allergic inflammatory disorders in various species of mammals...this system may be a target for treatment of immune-mediated and inflammatory disorders such as allergic skin diseases in dogs."[44]

SPINAL INJURY

Pets, like people, can suffer spinal injuries from accidents. In addition, many breeds, especially dog breeds, are predisposed to spinal injury from intervertebral disc disease. Although research looking at CBD's effect on recovery from spinal injury is fairly new, already researchers have found that rats treated with CBD following spinal cord injury have improved movement.[45] Administering cannabinoids soon after injury reduces pro-inflammatory cytokines, delays neuronal atrophy, and protects the myelin sheath surrounding the cord.[46]

VOMITING

Besides making a pet feel lousy, prolonged vomiting can cause dehydration and weight loss. Cannabinoids have been widely shown to have antiemetic (or anti-vomiting) effects. Although most research has been with THC and synthetic cannabinoids, CBD has also been shown to work in animal models.[47] "Preclinical research indicates that cannabinioids, including CBD, may be effective clinically for treating both nausea and vomiting produced by chemotherapy or other therapeutic treatments."[48]

The cannabinoid CBDA may be even more effective than CBD in reducing nausea and vomiting in animals.[49]

OTHER CONDITIONS

Besides these conditions, there is also limited evidence that cannabinoids may be helpful in the prevention or treatment of liver disease, kidney disease, and lower urinary tract infections. Much more research needs to be done to both uncover their full potential as well as sift out false leads. Cannabinoids are not miracle workers. They are not going to cure cancer—but they just may slow it or make it more bearable. Or maybe they actually *will* cure it in its early stages—we just don't know yet. There's no evidence of cannabinoids being helpful in another major disease of dogs, heart disease, or that they are able to combat common hereditary conditions such as progressive retinal atrophy, hip dysplasia or patellar luxation. But they may help alleviate anxiety from breathing or visual problems, or inflammation and pain from joint problems. Cannabinoids are not miracle workers—they won't fix everything—but for dogs with problems they do work on, they just may be miraculous.

CANNABINOIDS

	CBD	CBG	CBN	CBC	THCv	CBGA	CGCA	CBCA	THCA	CBDA	BCP
Relieves pain *Analgesic*	🐾			🐾	🐾	🐾					🐾
Suppresses appetite/Helps with weight loss *Anorectic*		🐾			🐾						🐾
Kills or slows bacteria growth *Antibacterial*	🐾							🐾			
Reduces blood sugar levels *Anti-diabetic*	🐾										
Reduces vomiting and nausea *Anti-emetic*	🐾									🐾	
Reduces seizures and convulsion *Anti-epileptic*	🐾									🐾	
Treats fungal infection *Antifungal*									🐾		
Reduces inflammation *Anti-inflammatory*	🐾					🐾			🐾	🐾	
Aids sleep *Anti-insomnia*			🐾								
Reduces risk of artery blockage *Anti-ischemic*	🐾										
Inhibits cell growth in tumors/cancer cells *Anti-proliferative*	🐾			🐾						🐾	
Treats psoriasis *Anti-psoriatic*	🐾										
Tranquilizing, used to manage psychosis *Antipsychotic*	🐾										
Suppresses muscle spasms *Antispasmodic*			🐾							🐾	
Relieves anxiety *Anxiolytic*			🐾								
Promotes bone growth *Bone Stimulant*					🐾					🐾	
Reduces contractions in the small intestines *Intestinal Anti-prokinetic*		🐾			🐾						
Protects nervous system degeneration *Neuroprotective*	🐾		🐾								

CLINICAL ENDOCANNABINOID DEFICIENCY (CEDC)

Cannabinoids are an essential part of lifelong nutrition to ensure optimal health. But what happens when a person or animal is deficient in normal levels? It's widely known that deficiencies in a variety of normal body chemicals are often found, and moreover, these deficiencies lead to suboptimal health or full-blown disease; for example, deficiencies in neurotransmitters can cause neural problems resulting in diseases affecting mood, cognition, and movement, among others. Likewise, naturally occurring endocannabinoid deficiencies almost surely exist. It would be foolish to believe that the body always makes sufficient levels of endocannabinoids to satisfy its needs, just as it doesn't always make enough of many other vitamins and nutrients it needs. When deficiencies of nutrients are discovered, drugs or supplements are used to take up the slack. In the case of endocannabinoid deficiency, we are fortunate that we can replace them with plant-derived cannabinoids. Could it be, for example, that people and pets who are susceptible to cancer (or anxiety or glaucoma or seizures) are cannabinoid deficient?

A 2004 article by Ethan B. Russo postulating endocannabinoid deficiencies behind several human conditions concluded, "Migraine, fibromyalgia, IBS and related conditions display common clinical, biochemical and pathophysiological patterns that suggest an underlying clinical endocannabinoid deficiency that may be suitably treated with cannabinoid medicines."[50]

In 2014, researchers revisited the earlier study. Not only did they verify the conclusions, they also added, "Subsequent research has confirmed that underlying endocannabinoid deficiencies indeed play a role in migraine, fibromyalgia, irritable bowel syndrome and a growing list of other medical conditions. Clinical experience is bearing this out. Further research and especially, clinical trials will further demonstrate the usefulness of medical cannabis. As legal barriers fall and scientific bias fades this will become more apparent."[51]

ENDOCANNABINOID DEFICIENCY SYNDROME

A 2014 veterinary journal postulated the occurrence of "endocannabinoid deficiency syndrome" in pets.

> As it turns out, the nervous, lymphatic and possibly other systems within the body already house cannabinoid receptors, making them already prepared to respond to both phyto- and endo-cannabinoids. Perhaps unsurprisingly, given the observed benefits of MMJ for epilepsy, the eCB system regulates neuronal excitability. When it falters, an "eCB deficiency syndrome" may result, associated not only with seizures but also with the onset of fibromyalgia, irritable bowel syndrome, migraine and other maladaptive states.

> In other words, while a normally functioning eCB system dampens neuronal excitation, its downregulation fosters neuronal hyperexcitability and dysfunction. In fact, many integrative approaches for epilepsy also affect eCB states, including acupuncture along with certain nutritional supplements, herbal medicines, dietary changes, and, of course, cannabis.[52]

As Dr. Russo concluded in his 2004 paper on CEDC, "...clinical cannabis has become a compass to what modern medicine fails to cure."[53]

CANNABINOIDS AND WELLNESS

It's apparent that cannabinoids are becoming vital tools in the fight against disease—but even more important is their value in maintaining health. This is especially true for middle-aged or senior pets. Modern advances in canine nutrition, medication, and therapies mean dogs are now living longer than ever. However, that often means they are living longer with degenerative health issues!

Cannabinoids prevent and combat common complaints of aging, including diminution of mental capacities, anxiety, lack of appetite, and inflammation and pain associated with arthritis. But beyond that, cannabinoids may simply make pets feel better, improving their comfort, mood, activity and appetite, so they feel and act like a younger version of themselves—and maybe even better! When your pet is more active, has better mental clarity, better muscle tone, better nutrition and maintains a proper weight, those factors contribute to better health, better quality of life, and longer life.

Even in younger pets, cannabinoids play an important role in maintaining homeostasis. Foremost among cannabinoids' benefits for healthy pets is their reduction of inflammation, as inflammation can bring on a host of problems including pain, autoimmune problems, cancer and arthritis. Cannabinoids are better used as a part of a holistic approach to pet health, not simply a therapy to turn to when things go wrong.

Unlike humans, pets can't tell you that they feel lethargic, depressed, or confused. Once owners notice such things, the condition is usually advanced. Nor can they go out and hunt for plants or foods that may contain nutrients missing in their diet. It's up to us to supply a balanced diet with any supplements their body may be lacking. Especially in light of the possibility of endo-cannabinoid deficiency syndrome, the prudent practice is to give our pets' bodies access to some of the most important natural compounds for their health and well-being: cannabinoids.

IN REVIEW:

- Fifty-plus years of medical research on cannabinoids have produced thousands of studies, revealing dozens of health applications in animals.
- CBD is the most well-known and often studied non-psychoactive cannabinoid and has been found to be non-toxic, with very few, if any, side effects.
- There are multiple cannabinoids in hemp that can potentially provide therapeutic benefit for dogs, including CBD, CBG, CBC and BCP.
- Endocannabinoid deficiency syndrome may be responsible for health issues in aging pets.
- Cannabinoids are not just for when your dog is sick or when pharmaceuticals fail. They are a beneficial component of daily nutrition for all pets.

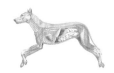

CHAPTER 4:

EFFECTIVE CANNABINOID PRODUCTS

I t seems like we should all be taking cannabinoid pills, and to some extent, we should. But you can't just eat a plant or swallow a pill to get the full benefits. For one, the health benefits of cannabis are not just due to cannabinoids alone. Cannabis plants have more than 500 chemical compounds in them, including cannabinoids, terpenes, and flavonoids, and many of them work together synergistically in an entourage effect. That's important. You can't just extract one cannabinoid, even CBD, and expect to get the same benefits you would from the whole plant.

In addition, cannabinoids also have to be properly extracted and activated from the acid forms present in raw hemp. In nature, cannabinoids are represented in their acid forms: CBDA, CBGA, CBCA, and so on. The reason historically that cannabis is cooked, smoked, or heated for therapeutic consumption is that the process of applying heat decarboxylates (converts) the acid forms to their activated counterparts: CBDA→CBD, CBGA→CBG,

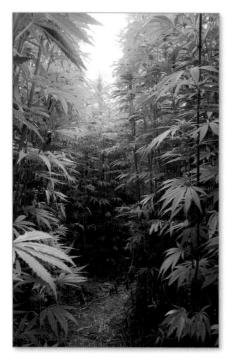

CBCA→CBC, and so forth. Since we wouldn't ask our dogs to smoke hemp, we have to ensure cannabinoids, terpenes, and flavonoids are extracted from the plant effectively.

In general, the acid forms of cannabinoids have different therapeutic effects from their activated counterparts, so it is important to maintain both for ultimate health; but for most applications, the activated components like CBD, CBC, and CBG are more significant than their acid counterparts CBDA, CBCA, and CBGA. The same temperatures that will activate cannabinoids will also destroy the volatile terpenes in the plant material that are vital to an entourage effect. This means extraction can't take place in one step.

The final form must be available to the dog's circulatory system. That's not as easy as it sounds.

Finally, if you wish to provide concentrated cannabinoids to your dog, there is only one legal and safe source: industrial hemp. Concentrated CBD and other cannabinoids are presently obtained from specialized industrial hemp oil extracts.

Hemp extracts are not created equal. The plant source, phytochemical diversity and ratios, extraction process and cannabinoid activation, quality checks, and product bioavailability make a huge difference when it comes to ensuring that the product not only contains activated cannabinoids, but also delivers them to your dog's endocannabinoid system.

SOURCE

Hemp plants absorb heavy metals, toxins, and even radiation from soil at a very high rate—so high that they are sometimes planted to reduce soil toxicity. While that's good for the environment, plants grown under such conditions are not a suitable source for edible products.

China produces about a quarter of all the hemp grown in the world, but a very high percentage of Chinese hemp is grown in soil contaminated with heavy metals and other pollutants. In some cases, the hemp is planted to detoxify the soil to ready it for food crops. Chinese hemp is the least expensive, but it is never acceptable.

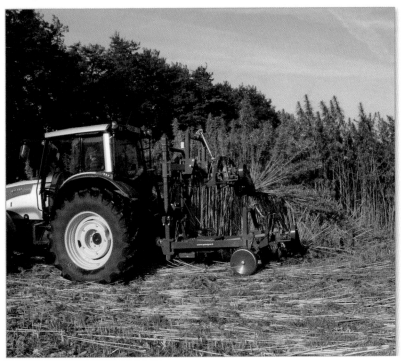

In the United States, according to the 2014 Farm Bill, a State department of agriculture may grow or cultivate industrial hemp if it satisfies two key requirements. First, the industrial hemp must be grown or cultivated "for purposes of research conducted under an agricultural pilot program or other agricultural or academic research." Second, the growing or cultivating of industrial hemp must be "allowed under the laws of the State in which such institution of higher education or State department of agriculture is located and such research occurs."[1] At least 23 states have enacted laws relating to industrial hemp, and several have begun producing experimental crops.

EXTRACTION

The method used to extract oils from hemp greatly affects the components of the final product. The simplest method, cold press extraction, is good for getting the seeds' nutrition and flavor but not for getting CBD and other cannabinoids. This method, which is much like the one used to produce olive oil, is used to produce hemp seed oil found in supermarkets. It doesn't concentrate the phytochemicals enough for any cannabinoid benefits.

The gold standard for producing a plant extract is that used by the essential oil industry, CO_2 (carbon dioxide) extraction.

At certain temperatures and pressures, CO_2 acts like a solvent without the dangers of actually being one. CO_2 extraction is widely considered the most effective and safest plant extraction method in the world; it's used, for example, to remove caffeine from coffee beans and to produce herbal supplements and essential oils. It's also the most expensive extraction method.

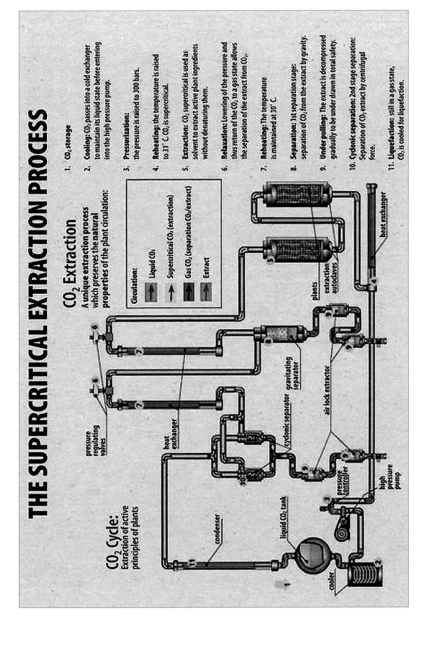

THE SUPERCRITICAL EXTRACTION PROCESS

CO₂ Extraction

A unique extraction process which preserves the natural properties of the plant circulation:

Circulation:

↑ Liquid CO₂

↑ Supercritical CO₂ (extraction)

↑ Gas CO₂ (separation CO₂/extract)

↑ Extract

1. CO₂ storage

2. **Cooling:** CO₂ passes into a cold exchanger to maintain its liquid state before entering into the high pressure pump.

3. **Pressurization:** the pressure is raised to 300 bars.

4. **Reheating:** the temperature is raised to 31°C. CO₂ is supercritical.

5. **Extraction:** CO₂ supercritical is used as solvent to extract active plant ingredients without denaturing them.

6. **Relaxation:** Lowering of the pressure and thus return of the CO₂ to a gas state allows the separation of the extract from CO₂.

7. **Reheating:** The temperature is maintained at 30°C.

8. **Separation:** 1st separation stage: separation of CO₂ from the extract by gravity.

9. **Under pulling:** The extract is decompressed gradually to be under drawn in total safety.

10. **Cyclonic separation:** 2nd stage separation: Separation of CO₂ extract by centrifugal force.

11. **Liquefaction:** still in a gas state, CO₂ is cooled for liquefaction.

CO₂ Cycle:

Extraction of active principles of plants

pressure regulating valves

heat exchanger

condenser

liquid CO₂ tank

cyclonic separator

gravitating separator

air lock extractor

plants

extraction autoclaves

heat exchanger

pressure controller

high pressure pump

cooler

High pressure and high temperature "supercritical" CO_2 extraction is effective at extracting larger molecules such as CBD and lipids like omega 3 and omega 6, chlorophyll, and waxes, but it damages most terpenes and heat-sensitive chemicals.

Low pressure and low temperature "subcritical" CO_2 extraction retains the essential oils, terpenes, and other sensitive chemicals, but it takes more time and produces much smaller yields.

"Full spectrum" CO_2 extractions combine the two processes. First, subcritical extraction is performed, followed by the supercritical extraction, and then both oil extracts are homogenized into one. This method preserves phytochemical diversity and enhances the entourage effect (the synergistic effect of multiple compounds). It provides for an array of both activated and acid form cannabinoids, and preserves the volatile terpenes and flavonoids in the oils. This is the process that provides whole-plant hemp extracts.

Most cannabis oils are the product of supercritical extraction only, rendering them completely lacking in terpenes and in secondary cannabinoids.

True full spectrum, whole-plant hemp oils are exceptionally rare.

	CANNABINOIDS											TERPENES						FLAVONOIDS		
	CBD	CBG	CBN	CBC	THCv	CBGA	CGCA	CBCA	THCA	CBDA	BCP	Alpha-Pinene	Humulene	Caryophylene Oxide	Limonene	Linalool	Myrcene	Apigenin	Cann flavin A	Quercetin
Relives pain / *Analgesic*	🐾	🐾	🐾	🐾		🐾						🐾	🐾				🐾	🐾		🐾
Suppresses appetite/Helps with weight loss / *Anorectic*					🐾															
Kills or slows bacteria growth / *Antibacterial*	🐾	🐾							🐾			🐾						🐾	🐾	
Reduces blood sugar levels / *Anti-diabetic*	🐾				🐾															
Reduces vomiting and nausea / *Anti-emetic*	🐾								🐾		🐾									
Reduces seizures and convulsion / *Anti-epileptic*	🐾		🐾													🐾				
Treats fungal infection / *Antifungal*	🐾	🐾		🐾		🐾		🐾	🐾		🐾	🐾	🐾	🐾	🐾		🐾	🐾	🐾	🐾
Reduces inflammation / *Anti-inflammatory*	🐾	🐾		🐾					🐾		🐾									
Aids sleep / *Anti-insomnia*			🐾																	
Reduces risk of artery blockage / *Anti-ischemic*	🐾																			
Inhibits cell growth in tumors/cancer cells / *Anti-proliferative*	🐾	🐾		🐾					🐾		🐾	🐾			🐾		🐾	🐾		🐾
Treats psoriasis / *Anti-psoriatic*	🐾																			
Tranquilizing, used to manage psychosis / *Antipsychotic*	🐾							🐾												
Suppresses muscle spasms / *Antispasmodic*	🐾	🐾		🐾		🐾					🐾									
Relieves anxiety / *Anxiolytic*	🐾														🐾	🐾	🐾			
Promotes bone growth / *Bone Stimulant*	🐾	🐾																		🐾
Reduces contractions in the small intestines / *Intestinal Anti-prokinetic*	🐾																			
Protects nervous system degeneration / *Neuroprotective*																				
Protects the GI Tract / *Gastroprotective*																		🐾	🐾	🐾

QUALITY CONTROL

It is important to conduct high performance liquid chromatography (HPLC) testing to determine the amounts of the various phytochemicals in each batch of raw material extract.

This enables batches to be blended to deliver consistent cannabinoid and terpene ratios and abundance. Screening for toxins and metals should also be done at this stage to ensure product safety.

PHYTOCHEMICAL DIVERSITY AND THE ENTOURAGE EFFECT

Effective hemp products require a diverse array of phytochemicals—not just CBD. As researchers continue to delve into the properties of cannabinoids, they are finding that every cannabinoid is different, each with its own benefits and effects on the body. Perhaps more importantly, they are finding that these compounds work additively and synergistically; that is, they interact to reinforce one another.

So while CBD may seem the star when it comes to medicinal cannabis, it has a host of supporting cast members that not only play their own roles, but allow the star to play off of them. The whole is greater than the sum of the parts; a drama with one character is seldom as effective as one with an entourage.

For example, not only does ß-caryophyllene (BCP) contribute its own anti-inflammatory properties, it also increases the uptake of CBD by the body.

TERPENES

It's not just the cannabinoids in hemp that work together. Cannabis plants also contain terpenes, organic compounds usually known for their strong fragrance and flavor. Terpenes are prevalent in hemp but also found in thousands of other plants besides cannabis. Terpenes are FDA-approved food additives and are common in human and animal diets. Terpenes can interact with cannabinoids in beneficial ways. For example, the terpene myrcene aids in allowing cannabinoids to cross the blood-brain barrier and is itself associated with antidepressant, anti-inflammatory, antimicrobial, anticarcinogen and antioxidant properties.[2] Humulene is a terpene with analgesic, antibacterial, anti-inflammatory, and antiproliferative properties.[3] Caryophyllene oxide is an antifungal. Linalool is an analgesic, anti-epileptic, antipsychotic, and anxiolitic. Limonene has antidepressant, antiepileptic, antipsychotic, and anxiolitic properties, and it stimulates the immune system and reduces gastroesophageal reflux.

Terpenes have been designated "generally recognized as safe" (GRAS) as a food additive by the U.S. Food and Drug Administration. See Appendix II for more details on terpenes, cannabinoids, and their entourage effects from the *British Journal of Pharmacology.*

FLAVONOIDS

In addition to terpenes, cannabis plants also contain flavonoids, plant metabolites known for their antioxidant and anti-inflammatory benefits. Quercetin is a type of flavonoid found in plant foods, including leafy greens, tomatoes, berries, and broccoli. It's also found in cannabis. Quercetin is technically considered a plant pigment, which is exactly why it's found in deeply colored, nutrient-packed fruits and vegetables. It is a potent antioxidant, and combinations of quercetin and other antioxidants probably work synergistically.[4] Quercetin is now largely utilized as a nutritional supplement to combat diabetes, obesity, circulatory dysfunction, inflammation, and mood disorders.[5]

Apigenin is a flavonoid found in fruits and vegetables including parsley, onions, oranges, tea, chamomile, wheat sprouts, and hemp, and "has been shown to possess remarkable anti-inflammatory, antioxidant and anti-carcinogenic properties."[6] Apigenin also demonstrates gastroprotective properties.[7] In 2016 it was reported that apigenin showed promising analgesic and anti-inflammatory activities.[8]

A flavonoid unique to cannabis, cannaflavin A, inhibits the inflammatory molecule PGE-2 thirty times more effectively than aspirin.[9]

ENTOURAGE EFFECT

The cannabinoids, terpenes and flavonoids in cannabis work together as a team, creating what is known as the entourage effect. The phrase was coined in 1999 by Dr. Ralph Mechoulam (the same scientist who first isolated THC and studied many non-psychoactive cannabinoids in the 1960s)[10] and elucidated by Dr. Ethan B. Russo in his seminal article on the topic.[11]

The entourage effect explains why synthetic versions of cannabinoids have often been disappointing compared to whole plant preparations. For example, Marinol, a prescription drug containing pure THC, has been found by physicians and patients alike to be a poor substitute for cannabis.

Pure CBD, too, is not nearly as effective alone as it is in the company of other compounds usually found with it in cannabis. Several studies have found that CBD in a cannabis plant extract is more effective than pure CBD. This includes its effect on slowing tumor proliferation and on pain and inflammation.[12]

Promoting a powerful entourage effect is the basis for the superiority of whole-plant extracts.

BIOAVAILABILITY

Why not just eat the whole hemp plant? For one, the quantity needed would be prohibitive; it would take pounds of raw hemp

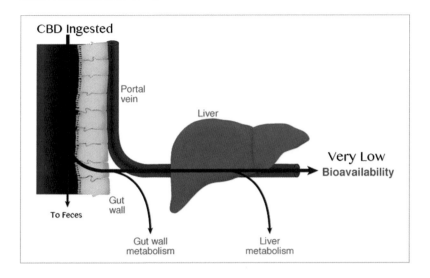

CBD Ingested

Portal vein

Liver

Very Low Bioavailability

To Feces

Gut wall

Gut wall metabolism

Liver metabolism

to produce the same amount of cannabinoids and terpenes present in one ounce of extracted product. In addition, the levels of cannabinoids and other components vary too much from plant to plant, so it would be impossible to standardize dosages. Further, the cannabinoids in raw plants are exclusively in their acid form, and they require activation. Finally, eating a plant is not an efficient way to deliver cannabinoids and other compounds into the bloodstream. This is what we mean when we talk about bioavailability.

Even when phytochemicals are properly extracted and activated from the plant source, there's a catch: when cannabis is eaten, the gastrointestinal tract and liver break down the CBD to metabolites (most notably 7-hydroxy-CBD and CBD-7-oic acid), which don't act as cannabinoids. Known as the hepatic first pass effect, it occurs because a product that is swallowed is absorbed by the digestive system and carried to the liver before it reaches the rest of the body. The liver then metabolizes the product, sometimes to such an extent that very little product is left to enter the circulatory system. This first pass effect can essentially neutralize the effects of many drugs and compounds, including the cannabinoids and terpenes. In fact, researchers have known as far back as 1988 that CBD is barely absorbed after oral administration to dogs.[13]

ORAL-MUCOSAL DELIVERY

The best solution is to bypass the gastrointestinal system and instead deliver the phytochemicals in a medium designed to dissolve in the mouth, which allows them to be absorbed directly into the bloodstream. This provides for rapid uptake of cannabinoids and very high bioavailability.

This is why the most successful pharmaceutical efforts into cannabinoids, such as GW Research Sativex products, are delivered via oral-mucosal spray, which allows for 10–15 times the bio-availability of digested products.[14]

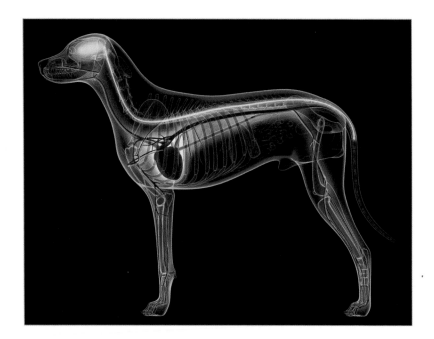

IN REVIEW:

A safe and effective cannabinoid product for your dog should:
- Use organic, quality screened hemp.
- Be produced using whole plant CO_2 extracts.
- Be screened for cannabinoid levels and toxins.
- Provide an abundance of diverse activated cannabinoids and terpenes, not just CBD.
- Effectively deliver those cannabinoids to your dog's endocannabinoid system (ECS) with high bioavailability.

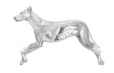

CHAPTER 5:

FIRSTHAND EXPERIENCES WITH CANNA-PET® HEMP PRODUCTS

Georgia, a Cavalier King Charles Spaniel, suffered from syringo-myelia, a serious and painful neurological disease caused by a malformation of the skull opening. Her owner, Kelly Conway, was desperate to find relief for Georgia. "This condition leaks spinal cord fluid and air pockets fill up her spine," said Conway. "She also has chronic dry eye, chronic ear infections and arthritis/hip dysplasia. My beautiful baby is a lemon."

Syringomelia tends to get progressively worse as the com-pressed spinal cord causes some parts of the body to feel as though they have "fallen asleep." It also causes itching, tingling and pain. "Georgia would bang her head, scratch, rub, and make her face bleed, trying to stop the pins and needles. Her neck and back hurt. She would bite her legs and do a helicopter scratch

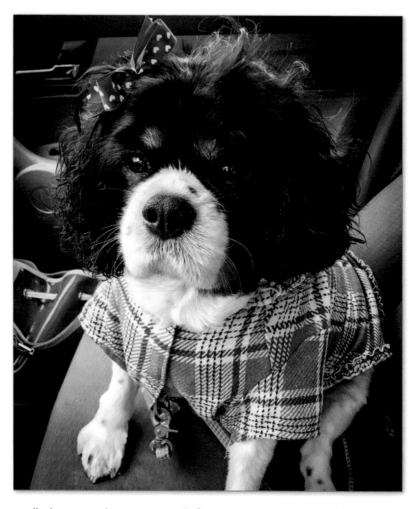

until she was almost crazy. " Georgia was already taking lots of Western medications, including gabapentin (Neurontin), Prilosec, tramadol and Novox (for hips and arthritis), plus she was getting acupuncture. When her veterinarian suggested Canna-Pet, Conway wasn't interested, as Georgia was already taking 12 pills a day. But when Conway broke her leg and had to give Georgia up for three months, Georgia's extreme separation anxiety added the impetus to give Canna-Pet a try. "The first two days, all Georgia did was sleep. I was scared. That wore off. After two weeks, I had a completely different dog."

"I truly expected nothing to change. I think it definitely takes the edge off of her pain, but the biggest change in Georgia was the reduction in anxiety. The decrease of anxiety decreased the head banging, scratching, and so on. The reduction of that behavior decreased the occurrence of eye and ear infections. My girl began to play with toys and other dogs, and I could hold her again. I can honestly say it was a mini-miracle for Georgia. She rarely takes tramadol for pain now. This past week has been bad due to the barometric pressure and constant rain in Philly, but she hasn't had a tramadol since well before Christmas. This is a big deal when discussing this painful condition."

Georgia was featured in a 2014 article about Canna-Pet on CNBC.[1] Conway has now been using Canna-Pet products for over two years with continued success and now has several other pets also using Canna-Pet products.

CHARLIE'S STORY

Charlie was a blind and deaf 14-year-old Pug with congestive heart failure—not exactly a dog with a future. His owners were giving him up, so Kristine Lauria took him in. She'd only had him a few months when he had his first seizures. The seizures started to come more often. "At first the medications worked, but then they couldn't control the seizures—he was having a grand mal weekly, then daily, then three or four a day. He no longer enjoyed life, and I had to face the decision whether to euthanize him. I remember it was on a Thursday. A friend suggested Canna-Pet; I figured what have I got to lose? I gave him the first dose Friday afternoon. Saturday he maybe seemed a bit different. I kept giving it to him, and Saturday evening he seemed to be walking more. By Sunday I remember thinking, 'This stuff is working!' He was rolling around,

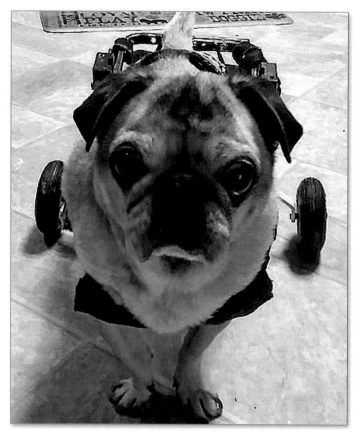

enjoying life! He still had seizures—but they were down to one a day or even less often—and his quality of life was back."

DEWEY'S STORY

Dewey's owners could no longer cope with the 12-year-old Pug, so they offered him for free on Craigslist. Fortunately, Lee Stevens of Harlee's Angels Rescue spotted the ad and brought him home. But he needed more than a home. "He had a hard time walking, and he just plain didn't enjoy life," recalls Stevens. So she tried Canna-Pet and gave Dewey a new lease on life. "Canna-Pet definitely helped him. His attitude is so much improved, he enjoys life much more, he's more alert. Before, he was dull-eyed and quiet; now he's bright-eyed and into everything. It's night and day!"

GLADYS'S STORY

Harlee's Angels specializes in Pugs in need, so when another rescue group was ready to give up on Gladys, they contacted Lee Stevens. Gladys suffered brain injuries when she'd been hit by a car and left on the roadside. The brain injuries caused intractable cluster seizures that weren't responding to medication. Says Stevens: "Within 24 hours of starting Canna-Pet, she quit seizing. Now she has a seizure about once a week—a huge improvement!"

MORE HARLEE'S ANGELS STORIES

Lee Stevens has treated several other dogs at Harlee's Angels with Canna-Pet:

Yet another Pug, 18-year-old Olaf, was found in a blizzard, almost frozen. He had mobility problems and anxiety issues. "Canna-Pet has helped his quality of life and especially helped with his anxiety," says Stevens.

Bruiser, a Saint Bernard, had joint problems. Stevens: "The Canna-Pet helped with inflammation, and in turn, he's walking better."

Marlee, another Saint Bernard, has elbow dysplasia. "She was in pain, and whined all the time," recalls Stevens, "but within a week of starting Canna-Pet, she was no longer whining."

Stevens cautions that it's not a miracle cure: "I don't think it helped with congestive heart failure, for example. It didn't make blind dogs see or deaf dogs hear! But it helps immensely with their quality of life, making them less painful and less anxious. It makes a huge difference."

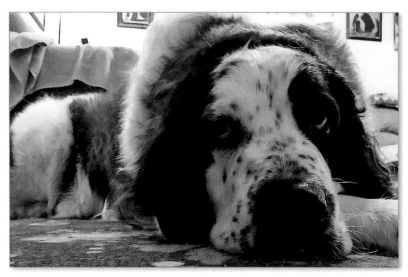

MILES'S STORY

Donna Butler uses Canna-Pet for her dog Miles, who is paralyzed from the waist down. He lost mobility in his back legs after being diagnosed with degenerative myelopathy, the equivalent of ALS (Lou Gehrig's disease) in humans.

"He was starting to get real anxious," recalls Butler. "He was starting to react to loud noise in a way that he never had."

Butler asked her veterinarian for something that would calm Miles's anxiety. Her doctor, Angie Stamm, DVM, went with Canna-Pet as a natural remedy.

"He's just much more content," Butler says.[2] "He's just much more stable."

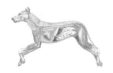

CHAPTER 6:

THE THERAPEUTIC HEMP INDUSTRY FOR PETS AS OF AUGUST 2016

When choosing a cannabis product, you should choose one that is made specifically for pets. Dogs and cats have a lower tolerance for THC and may be more sensitive to miniscule amounts a human would not notice.

Several companies now offer cannabis products for pets. As these are marketed as supplements, not drugs, there's not as much oversight as might otherwise be desirable. Buyers should be cautious of upstart companies.

The pioneer is the field is a Seattle company, Canna-Pet®. They claim to be (and that claim appears to be true) the only provider with a multi-year product track record, established research connections with major veterinary universities, third-party published data on their products, and acceptance by major pet insurers like Trupanion and Petplan (with proper riders for herbal therapy). They remain the only company to have achieved formal registration for their cannabinoid pet products with the United States Patent and Trademark Office (USPTO).

The company assures that its products meet the recommendations for manufacture outlined in Chapter 4, using Industrial hemp, full-spectrum CO_2 extraction, high-performance liquid chromatography (HPLC) testing, phytochemical diversity, and oral-mucosal delivery for best bioavailability. The products contain over two dozen cannabinoids, terpenes, and flavonoids, including CBD, ß-caryophyllene, CBC, CBG, limonene, α-pinene, and linalool. All production occurs in the United States.

Canna-Pet appears to have many satisfied customers, judging from online testimonials as well as the ones cited in this book. The company offers a money-back satisfaction guarantee and has made available a discount to readers:

**Via the Canna-Pet.com website,
any new customers who use coupon code**

CannabisScience

**will receive 30% off their first order, and a
portion of the proceeds will also be donated
to the AKC Canine Health Foundation and
the San Diego Humane Society.**

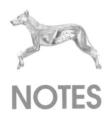

NOTES

CHAPTER 1:

1. Historical Timeline. (2013, August 13). Retrieved from http://medicalmarijuana.procon.org/view.timeline.php?timelineID=000026

2. Gupta, S. (2013, August 8). Why I changed my mind on weed. Retrieved from http://www.cnn.com/2013/08/08/health/gupta-changed-mind-marijuana/

3. Gupta, S. (2014, March 11). Medical marijuana and the "entourage effect." Retrieved from http://www.cnn.com/2014/03/11/health/gupta-marijuana-entourage/

4. Robinson, N. (2015, September 29). The Latest on Cannabis and Hemp for Pets. *Veterinary Practice News*. Retrieved from http://www.veterinarypracticenews.com/the-latest-on-cannabis-and-hemp-for-pets/

CHAPTER 2

1. Sula, B. (1975) Early Diffusion and Folk Uses of Hemp in Cannabis and Culture. In V.D. Rubin (Eds.) Cannabis and Culture (pp. 39-49). The Hague: Mouton.

2. Butrica, J. (2002) The Medical Use of Cannabis Among the Greeks and Romans. *Journal of Cannabis Therapeutics 2*(2), 51. Retrieved from http://www.tandfonline.com/doi/abs/10.1300/J175v02n02_04#.VzTWJyMrKfU

3.   North, C. (2013, October 28) Cannabis: India 1500 BC. Retrieved from Inity Weekly website: http://inityweekly.com/mmj-india-1000-bc/

4.   Sulak, D. (n.d.) Introduction to the Endocannabinoid System. Retrieved from the NORML website: http://norml.org/library/item/ introduction-to-the-endocannabinoid-system)

5.   McPartland, J.M. & Guy,G.W. (2006) The evolution of Cannabis and coevolution with the cannabinoid receptor—a hypothesis. In Guy, et al. (Eds.), *The Medicinal Uses of Cannabinoids*. McPartland, J.M. et al, (2006) Evolutionary origins of the endocannabinoid system." *Gene 370*, 64-74.

6.   McPartland, J.M., Agraval, J., Gleeson, D., Heasman, K., & Glass, M. (2006). Cannabinoid receptors in invertebrates. *Journal for Evolutionary Biology, European Society for Evolutionary Biology, 19*(2), 366-73.

7.   Hampson, A.J., Axelrod, J., & Grimaldi, Maurizio. (2003). U.S. Patent No. 6,630,507. U.S. Patent and Trademark Office. Retrieved from http://patft.uspto.gov/netacgi/nph-Parser?Se ct1=PTO1&Sect2=HITOFF&d=PALL&p=1&u=%2Fnetahtm l%2FPTO%2Fsrchnum.htm&r=1&f=G&l=50&s1=6630507. PN.&OS=PN/6630507&RS=PN/6630507

8.   Gertsch, J., Leonti, M., Raduner, S., Racz, I., Chen, J.Z., Xie, X.Q., Altmann,K.H.,… & A. Zimmer. (2008). Beta-caryophyllene is a dietary cannabinoid. *Proceedings of the National Academy of Sciences, 105*(26), 9099-104. Retrieved from doi: 10.1073/pnas.0803601105. Epub 2008 Jun 23.

9.   Gertsch, J., Leontini, M., Raduner, S., Racz, I., Chen, J.Z., Xie, X.Q., … Zimmer, A. (2008). Beta-caryophyllene is a dietary cannabinoid. *Proceedings of the National Academy of Sciences,* USA 105(26), 9099-104. Retrieved from http://www.ncbi.nlm.nih.gov/pubmed/18574142; Lovett, R.A. (2008, June 24). Marijuana Has Anti-Inflammatory That Won't Get You High. Retrieved from National Geographic websitehttp:// news.nationalgeographic.com/news/2008/06/080624-marijuana.html

CHAPTER 3

1.   U.S. National Library of Medicine and National Institutes of Health. Retrieved from http://www.ncbi.nlm.nih.gov/ pubmed/?term=cannbinoids

2. U.S. National Library of Medicine and National Institutes of Health. Retrieved from http://www.ncbi.nlm.nih.gov/pubmed/?term=cannabidiol

3. Izzo, A.A. (2009). "Non-psychotropic plant cannabinoids: new therapeutic opportunities from an ancient herb." *Trends in Pharmacological Sciences, 30*(10), 515-27.

4. Bergamaschi, M.M., Queiroz, R.H., Zuardi, A.W., & Crippa, J.A. (2011). Safety and side effects of cannabidiol, a Cannabis sativa constituent. *Current Drug Safety, 6*(4), 237-49. Retrieved from http://www.ncbi.nlm.nih.gov/pubmed/22129319

5. Parker, L.A., Burton, P., Sorge, R.E., Yakiwchuk, C., & Mechoulam, R. (2004). Effect of low doses of delta9-tetrahydrocannabinol and cannabidiol on the extinction of cocaine-induced and amphetamine-induced conditioned place preference learning in rats. *Psychopharmacology, 175*(3), 360-66. Retrieved from http://www.ncbi.nlm.nih.gov/pubmed/15138755; Prud'homme, M., Cata, R., & Jutras-Aswad, D. (2015, May 21). Cannabidiol as an Intervention for Addictive Behaviors: A Systematic Review of the Evidence. *Substance Abuse, 9,* 33-38. Retrieved from http://www.ncbi.nlm.nih.gov/pmc/articles/PMC4444130/; Ren, Y., Whittard, J., Higuera-Matas, A., Morris, C.V., & Hurd, Y.L. (2009 November 25). Cannabidiol, a nonpsychotropic component of cannabis, inhibits cue-induced heroin-seeking and normalizes discrete mesolimbic neuronal disturbances. *Journal of Neuroscience, 29*(47), 14764-14769. Retrieved from http://www.ncbi.nlm.nih.gov/pmc/articles/PMC2829756/#R21

6. Tambaro, S. & Bortolato, M. (2012). Cannabinoid-related agents in the treatment of anxiety disorders: current knowledge and future perspectives. *Recent Patents on CNS Drug Discovery, 7*(1), 25-40. Retrieved from http://www.ncbi.nlm.nih.gov/pmc/articles/PMC3691841/

7. de Mello Schier, A.R., de Oliveira Ribeiro, N.P., de Oliveira e Silva, A.C., Cecilio Hallak, J.E., Crippa, J.A.S., Nardi, A.E., & Zuardi, A.W. (2012). Cannabidiol, a Cannabis sativa constituent, as an anxiolytic drug. *Revista Brasileira de Psiquiatria, 34*(1). Retrieved from http://www.scielo.br/scielo.php?pid=S1516-44462012000500008&script=sci_arttext

8. Ramirez, B., Blazquez, C. Gomez del Pulgar, T., Guzman, M., & de Ceballos, Maria L. (2005). Prevention of Alzheimer's Disease Pathology by Cannabinoids: Neuroprotection Mediated by Blockade of Microglial Activation. *The Journal of Neuroscience, 25*(8), 1904-1913. Retrieved from http://www.jneurosci.org/content/25/8/1904.full

9. Karl, T., Cheng, D., Garner, B., & Arnold, J.C. (2012). The therapeutic potential of the endocannabinoid system for Alzheimer's disease. *Expert Opinion on Therapeutic Targets, 16*(4), 407-20. Retrieved from http://www.ncbi.nlm.nih.gov/pubmed/22448595; Iuvone, T., Esposito, G., Esposito, R., Santamaria, R., DiRosa, M., & Izzo, A.A. (2004). Neuroprotective effect of cannabidiol, a non-psychoactive component from Cannabis sativa, on beta-amyloid-induced toxicity in PC12 cells. *Journal of Neurochemistry, 89*(1), 134-41. Retrieved from http://www.ncbi.nlm.nih.gov/pubmed/15030397

10. Malfait, A.M., Gallily, R., Sumariwalla, P.F., Malik, A.S., Andreakos, E., Mechoulam, R., & Feldmann, M. (2000). The nonpsychoactive cannabis constituent cannabidiol is an oral anti-arthritic therapeutic in murine collagen-induced arthritis. *Proceedings of the National Academy of Sciences,* USA 97(17), 9561-9566. Retrieved from http://www.ncbi.nlm.nih.gov/pmc/articles/PMC16904/

11. Massi, P., Vaccani, A. & Parolaro, D. (2006). Cannabinoids, immune system and cytokine network. *Current Pharmaceutical Design, 12*(24), 3135-46. Retrieved from http://www.ncbi.nlm.nih.gov/pubmed/16918439

12. Venkatesh, L. Hegede, Tomar, S., Jackson, A., Rao, R., Yang, X., Singh, U. ... Nagarkatti, M. (2013). Distinct microRNA expression profile and targeted biological pathways in functional myeloid-derived suppressor cells induced by Δ9-Tetrahydrocannabinol in vivo: Regulation of CCAAT/enhancer binding protein alpha by micro RNA-690. *Journal of Biological Chemistry.* Retrieved from http://www.jbc.org/content/early/2013/11/07/jbc.M113.503037.abstract?sid=7da5b2a0-9940-4ea3-90b4-eed1d9107a51

13. Bab, I., Zimmer, A., & Melamed, E. (2009). Cannabinoids and the skeleton: from marijuana to reversal of bone loss. *Annals of Medicine, 41*(8), 560-67. Retrieved from http://www.ncbi.nlm.nih.gov/pubmed/19634029; http://www.ncbi.nlm.nih.gov/pubmed/23181053

14. Kogan, N.M., Melamed, E., Wasserman, E., Raphael, B., Breuer, A., Stok, K. ... Bab, I. (2015). Cannabidiol, a Major Non-Psychotropic Cannabis Constituent Enhances Fracture Healing and Stimulates Lysyl Hydroxylase Activity in Osteoblasts. *Journal of Bone and Mineral Research 30*(10), 1905-1913. Retrieved from http://onlinelibrary.wiley.com/doi/10.1002/jbmr.2513/pdf

15. National Cancer Institute. (2015, April 10). Complementary and Alternative Medicine for Health Professionals. Rockville, MD. Retrieved

from http://www.cancer.gov/about-cancer/treatment/cam/hp/cannabis-pdq#section/_7

16. Freimuth, N., Ramer, R. & Hinz, B. (2010). Antitumorigenic effects of cannabinoids beyond apoptosis. *Journal of Pharmacology and Experimental Therapeutics, 332*(2), 336-44. Retrieved from http://www.ncbi.nlm.nih.gov/pubmed/19889794

17. Kogan, N.M., (2005). Cannabinoids and Cancer. *Mini-Reviews in Medicinal Chemistry, 5,* 941-52. Retrieved from http://theroc.us/images/Cannabinoids%20and%20Cancer.pdf

18. Aviello, G., Romano, B., & Izzo, A.A. (2008). Cannabinoids and gastrointestinal motility: animal and human studies. *European Review for Medical and Pharmacological Sciences, 12*(1), 81-93. Retrieved from http://www.ncbi.nlm.nih.gov/pubmed/18924447

19. Sabo, A., Horvat, O., Stilinovic, N., Berenil, J., & Vukmirovic, S. (2013). Industrial hemp decreases intestinal motility stronger than indian hemp in mice. *European Review for Medical and Pharmacological Sciences, 17*(4), 486-90. Retrieved from http://www.ncbi.nlm.nih.gov/pubmed/23467947

20. Carter, G.T., Abood, M.E., Aggarwal, S.K., & Weiss, M.D. (2010). Cannabis and amyotrophic lateral sclerosis: hypothetical and practical applications, and a call for clinical trials. *American Journal of Hospice and Palliative Care, 27*(5): 347-56. Retrieved from http://www.ncbi.nlm.nih.gov/pubmed/20439484

21. Ngueta, G., Belanger, R., Lauan-Sidi, E.A., & Lucas, M. (2014, December 13). Cannabis use in relation to obesity and insulin resistance in the Inuit population. *Obesity 23*(2), 290-95. Retrieved from http://onlinelibrary.wiley.com/doi/10.1002/oby.20973/abstract

22. Weiss, L., Zeira, M., Reich, S., Har-Noy, M., Mechoulam, R., Slavin, S., & Gallily, R. (2006). Cannabidiol lowers incidence of diabetes in non-obese diabetic mice. *Autoimmunity, 39*(2), 143-51. Retrieved from http://www.ncbi.nlm.nih.gov/pubmed/16698671

23. CBD compound in cannabis could treat diabetes, researchers suggest. (2015 April 24). Retrieved from the Diabetes.co.uk website http://www.diabetes.co.uk/news/2015/Apr/cbd-compound-in-cannabis-could-treat-diabetes,-researchers-suggest-95335970.html

24. Wargent, E.T., Zaibi, M.S., Silvestri, C., Hislop, D.C., Stocker, C.J., Stott, C.G., Guy, G.W. ... Cawthorne, M.A. (2013). The cannabinoid

tetrahydrocannabivarin (THCV) ameliorates insulin sensitivity in two mouse models of obesity. *Nutrition and Diabetes, 3*(5), e68. Retrieved from http://www.ncbi.nlm.nih.gov/pmc/articles/PMC3671751/

25. Hampson, A.J., Axelrod, J., & Grimaldi, M. (2003). US6630507. Retrieved from http://www.google.com/patents/US6630507

26. Colasanti, B.K. (2009). A Comparison of the Ocular and Central Effects of Tetrahydrocannabinol and Cannabigerol. *Journal of Ocular Pharmacology and Therapeutics, 6*(4), 259-69. Retrieved from http://online.liebertpub.com/doi/abs/10.1089/jop.1990.6.259

27. Appendino, G., Gibbons, S., Giana, A. Pagani,A., Grassi, G., Starvi, M., Smith, E., & Rahman, M.M. (2008). Antibacterial cannabinoids from Cannabis sativa: a structure-activity study. *Journal of Natural Products, 71*(8), 1427-30. Retrieved from http://www.ncbi.nlm.nih.gov/pubmed/18681481

28. Van Klingeren, B., & Ten Ham, M. (1976). Antibacterial activity of delta9-tetrahydrocannabinol and cannabidiol. *Antonie Van Leeuwenhoek, 42*(1-2), 9-12. Retrieved from http://www.ncbi.nlm.nih.gov/pubmed/1085130

29. Turner, C.E., & Elsohly, M.A. (1981). Biological activity of cannabichromene, its homologs and isomers. *Journal of Clinical Pharmacology, 21*(8-9 Suppl), 283S-291S. Retrieved from http://www.ncbi.nlm.nih.gov/pubmed/7298870

30. Edwards, T. (2005) Inflammation, Pain, and Chronic Disease: An Integrative Approach to Treatment and Prevention. *Alternative Therapies, 11*(6), 20-27.

31. Nagarkatti, P., Pandey, R., Rieder, S.A.,Hegde, V.L., & Nagarkatti, M. (2009). Cannabinoids as novel anti-inflammatory drugs. *Future Medicinal Chemistry 1*(7), 1333-1349. Retrieved from http://www.ncbi.nlm.nih.gov/pmc/articles/PMC2828614/

32. Ngueta, G., Belanger, R.E., Laouan-Sidi, E.A., & Lucas, M. (2015). Cannabis use in relation to obesity and insulin resistance in the Inuit population. *Obesity 2*, 290-95. Retrieved from http://www.ncbi.nlm.nih.gov/pubmed/25557382

33. Rodondi, N., Pletcher, M.J., Liu, K., Hulley, S.B., & Sidney, S. (2006) Marijuana use, diet, body mass index, and cardiovascular risk factors (from the CARDIA study). *The*

American Journal of Cardiology, 98(4), 478-84. Retrieved from http://www.ncbi.nlm.nih.gov/pubmed/16893701/

34. Nardo, M., Casarotto, PI, Gomes, F.V., & Guimaraes, F.S. (2014). Cannabidiol reverses the mCPP-induced increase in marble-burying behavior. *Fundamental and Clinical Pharmacology, 28*(5), 544-50. Retrieved from http://onlinelibrary.wiley.com/doi/10.1111/fcp.12051/ abstract

35. Khasabova, I., Khasabov, S., Paz, J., Harding-Rose, C., Simone, D.A., & Seybold, V.S. (2012). Cannabinoid type-1 receptor reduces pain and neurotoxicity produced by chemotherapy. *The Journal of Neuroscience, 32*(20), 7091-7101. Retrieved from http://www.ncbi.nlm.nih.gov/pmc/ articles/PMC3366638/

36. Khasabova, I.A., Gielissen, J., Chandiramani, A., Harding-Rose, C., Odeh, D.A., Simone, D.A., & Seybold, V.S. (2011). CB1 and CB2 receptor agonists promote analgesia through synergy in a murine model of tumor pain. *Behavioural Pharmacology, 22*(5-6), 607-16. Retrieved from http://www.ncbi.nlm.nih.gov/pubmed/21610490?dopt=Abstract

37. Curto-Reyes, V., Llames, S., Hidalgo, A., Menendez, L., & Baamonde, A. (2010). Spinal and peripheral analgesic effects of the CB2 cannabinoid receptor agonist AM 1241 in two models of bone cancer-induced pain. *British Journal of Pharmacology, 160*(3), 561-573. Retrieved from http:// www.ncbi.nlm.nih.gov/pmc/articles/PMC2931557/?tool=pubmed; Lozano-Ondoua, A.N., Wright, C., Vardanya, A., King, T., Largent-Milnes, T.M., Nelson, M., … Vanderah, T.W. (2010). A cannabinoid 2 recepton agonist attenuates bone cancer-induced pain and bone loss. *Life Sciences, 86*(17-18), 646-53. Retrieved from http://www.ncbi.nlm.nih. gov/pubmed/20176037

38. Wallace, Robyn. (2004). Cannabinoids: Defending the Epileptic Brain. *Epilepsy Currents, 4*(3), 93-95. Retrieved from http://www.ncbi.nlm. nih.gov/pmc/articles/PMC1176332/; Hill, A.J., Mercier, M.S., Hill, T.D., Glyn, S.E., Jones, N.A., Yamasaki, Y., Futamura, T. … Whalley, B.J. (2012). Cannabidivarin is anticonvulsant in mouse and rat. *British Journal of Pharmacology, 167*(8), 1629-42. Retrieved from http://www.ncbi.nlm. nih.gov/pubmed/22970845

39. Jones, N.A., Glyn, S.E., Akiyama, S., Hill, T.D., Hill, A.J., Weston, S.E., … Williams, C.M. (2012). Cannabidiol exerts anti-convulsant effects in animal models of temporal lobe and partial seizures. *Seizure, 21*(5), 344-52. Retrieved from http://www.ncbi.nlm.nih.gov/pubmed/22520455

40. Charlotte's Web CNN Special Dr. Sanjay Gupta. (2015, January 5). [Video file]. Retrieved from https://www.youtube.com/watch?v=PKvbaliLKvE

41. Stander, S., Reinhardt, H.W., & Luger, T.A. (2006). Topical cannabinoid agonists. An effective new possibility for treating chronic pruritus. Hautarzt 57(9), 801-07. Retrieved from http://www.ncbi.nlm.nih.gov/pubmed/16874533

42. Karsak, M., Gaffal, E., Date, R., Wang-Eckhardt, L., Rehnelt, J., Petrosino, S., ... Zimmer, A. (2007). *Science, 316*(5830), 1494-97. Retrieved from http://www.ncbi.nlm.nih.gov/pubmed/17556587

43. Biro, T., Balazs, T., Hasko, G., Paus, R., & Pacher, P. (2009, July 14). The endocannabinoid system of the skin in health and disease: novel perspectives and therapeutic opportunities. *Trends in Pharmacological Sciences, 30*(8), 411-420. Retrieved from http://www.ncbi.nlm.nih.gov/pmc/articles/PMC2757311/

44. Campora, L., Miragliotta, V., Ricci, E., Cristino, L., Di Marzo, V., Albanese, F., Federica Della Valle, M., & Abramo, F. (2012). Cannabinoid receptor type 1 and 2 expression in the skin of healthy dogs and dogs with atopic dermatitis. *American Journal of Veterinary Research, 73*(7), 988-95. Retrieved from http://www.ncbi.nlm.nih.gov/pubmed/22738050

45. Kwiatkosti, M., Guimaraes, F.S., & Del-Bel, E. (2012). Cannabidiol-treated rats exhibited higher motor score after cryogenic spinal cord injury. *Neurotoxicity Research, 21*(3), 271-80. Retrieved from http://www.ncbi.nlm.nih.gov/pubmed/21915768

46. Latini, L., Bisicchia, E., Sasso, V., Chiurchiu, V., Cavallucci, V., Molinari, M., Maccarrone, M., & Viscomi, M.T. (2014, September 4). Cannabinoid CB2 receptor (CB2R) stimulation delays rubrospinal mitochondrial-dependent degeneration and improves functional recovery after spinal cord hemisection by ERK1/2 inactivation. *Cell Death and Disease 5*, e1404. Retrieved from http://www.nature.com/cddis/journal/v5/n9/full/cddis2014364a.html; http://www.ncbi.nlm.nih.gov/pubmed/23152849

47. Arevalo-Martin, A., Garcia-Ovejero, D., Sierra-Palomares, Y., Paniagua-Torija, B., Gonzalez-Gil, I., Ortega-Gutierrez, S., & Molina-Holgado, E. (2012, November 13). Early endogenous activation of CB1 and CB2 receptors after spinal cord injury is a protective response involved in spontaneous recovery. *PloS One, 7*(11), e49057. Retrieved from http://www.ncbi.nlm.nih.gov/pubmed/13680081?dopt=Abstract

48. Parker, L.A., Rock, E.M., & Limebeer, C.L. (2011). Regulation of nausea and vomiting by cannabinoids. *British Journal of Pharmacology, 163*(7), 1411-22. Retrieved from http://www.ncbi.nlm.nih.gov/pubmed/21175589

49. Bolognini, D., Rock, E.M., Cluny, N.L., Cascio, M.G., Limebeer, C.L., Duncan, M., Stott, C.G., ... Pertwee, R.G. (2013). Cannabidiolic acid prevents vomiting in Suncus murinus and nausea-induced behaviour in rats by enhancing 5-HT1A receptor activation, *British Journal of Pharmacology, 168*(6), 1456-70. Retrieved from http://www.ncbi.nlm.nih.gov/pubmed/23121618

50. Russo, E.B. (2004). Clinical Endocannabinoid Deficiency (CECD): Can this Concept Explain Therapeutic Benefits of Cannabis in Migraine, Fibromyalgia, Irritable Bowel Syndrome and other Treatment-Resistant Conditions? *Neuroendocrinology Letters, 25*(1/2), 31-39. Retrieved from http://www.nel.edu/pdf_/25_12/NEL251204R02_Russo_.pdf

51. Smith, S.C., & Wagner, M.S. (2014). Clinical endocannabinoid deficiency (CECD) revisited: can this concept explain the therapeutic benefits of cannabis in migraine, fibromyalgia, irritable bowel syndrome and other treatment-resistant conditions? *Neuroendocrinology Letters, 35*(3), 198-201. Retrieved from http://www.ncbi.nlm.nih.gov/pubmed/24977967

52. Robinson, N. Cannabis for Intractable Epilepsy. Veterinary Practice News. Retrieved from http://www.veterinarypracticenews.com/Cannabis-for-Intractable-Epilepsy/

53. Russo, E.B. (2008). Clinical Endocannabinoid Deficiency (CECD): Can this Concept Explain Therapeutic Benefits of Cannabis in Migraine, Fibromyalgia, Irritable Bowel Syndrome and other Treatment-Resistant Conditions? *Neuroendocrinology Letters 29*(2), 192-200. Retrieved from http://cannabisclinicians.org/wp-content/uploads/2014/07/Russo-Clinical-endocannabinoid-deficiency.pdf

CHAPTER 4

1. 7 USC § 7606(a).

2. Russo, E. (2011 July 12). Taming THC: potential cannabis synergy and phytocannabinoid-terpenoid entourage effects. *British Journal of Pharmacology, 163*(7), 1-21. Retrieved from http://onlinelibrary.wiley.com/doi/10.1111/j.1476-5381.2011.01238.x/pdf

3. Colbert, M. (2014, November 20). Terpene Profile: Humulene. Retrieved from The Leaf Online website: http://theleafonline.com/c/science/2014/11/terpene-profile-humulene/

4. Middleton, E. Jr., Kandaswami, C., & Theoharides, T.C. (2000) The effects of plant flavonoids on mammalian cells: implications for inflammation, heart disease, and cancer. *Pharmacological Reviews, 52,* 673-751. Retrieved from http://ajcn.nutrition.org/content/78/3/570S.full#ref-6

5. D'Andrea, G. (2015). Quercetin: A flavonol with multifaceted therapeutic applications. *Fitoterapia, 106,* 256–271. Retrieved from http://www.sciencedirect.com/science/article/pii/S0367326X15300927; Narenjkar, J. (2011) The Effect of the Flavonoid Quercetin on Pain Sensation in Diabetic Rats. *Basic and Clinical NeuroScience, 2*(3), 51-57. Retrieved from http://bcn.iums.ac.ir/files/site1/user_files_c424bc/admin-A-10-1-64-22ffb5b.pdf

6. Patel, D., Shukla, S., & Gupta, S. (2007). Apigenin and cancer chemoprevention: progress, potential and promise (review)" *International Journal of Oncology, 30*(1), 233-45. Retrieved from http://www.ncbi.nlm.nih.gov/pubmed/17143534

7. Pirvu, L., Dragomir, C., Schiopu, S., & Mihul, S.C. Vegetal extracts with gastroprotective activity. (2012). *Romanian Biotechnological Letters, 17*(2). Retrieved from http://www.rombio.eu/rbl2vol17/14.pdf

8. El Shoubaky, G.A., Abdel Damin, M.M., Mansour, M.H., & Salem, E.A. (2016, February 16). Isolation and Identification of a Flavone Apigenin from marine Red Alga Acanthophora spicifera with Antinociceptive and Anti-Inflammatory Activities. *Journal of Experimental Neuroscience, 10,* 21-29. Retrieved from http://www.ncbi.nlm.nih.gov/pubmed/26917974

9. Barrett, M.L, Scutt, A.M., & Evans, F.J. (1986) Cannflavin A and B, prenylated flavones from Cannabis sativa L. *Experientia, 42,* 452–3. Retrieved from http://www.ncbi.nlm.nih.gov/pubmed/3754224

10. Gupta, S. (2014, March 11) Medical marijuana and "the entourage effect." [Video file]. Retrieved from http://www.cnn.com/2014/03/11/health/gupta-marijuana-entourage/

11. Russo, E. (2011). Taming THC: potential cannabis synergy and phytocannabinoid-terpenoid entourage effects. *British Journal of Pharmacology, 163*(7), 1344–1364. Retrieved from http://www.ncbi.nlm.nih.gov/pmc/articles/PMC3165946/

12. Romano, B., Borrelli, F., Pagano, E., Cascio, M.G., Pertwee, R.G., & Izzo, A.A. (2014). Inhibition of Colon Carcinogenesis by a Standardized Cannabis Sativa Extract with High Content of Cannabidiol. *Phytomedicine, 21,* 631-639. Retrieved from http://www.ncbi.nlm.nih.gov/pubmed/24373545; Gallily, R., Yekhtin, Z. & Hanus, L.O. (2015). Overcoming the Bell-Shaped Dose-Response of Cannabidiol by Using Cannabisi Extract Enriched in Cannabidiol. *Pharmacology and Pharmacy, 6*(2), 75-85. http://www.scirp.org/journal/PaperInformation.aspx?PaperID=53912#.VVNpXCjR5US

13. Samara, E., Bialer, M., & Mechoulam, R. (1988). Pharmacokinetics of cannabidiol in dogs. *Drug metabolism and disposition: the biological fate of chemicals, 16*(3), 469-72. Retrieved from http://www.ncbi.nlm.nih.gov/pubmed/2900742

14. Karschner, E., Darwin, W.D., Goodwin, R.S., Wright, S., & Huestis, M.A. (2011) Plasma Cannabinoid Pharmocokinetics following Controlled Δ9-Tetrahydrocannabinol and Oromucosal Cannabis Extract Administration. *Clinical Chemistry, 57*(1), 66-75. Retrieved from http://www.ncbi.nlm.nih.gov/pmc/articles/PMC3717338/

CHAPTER 5

1. Weisbaum, H. (2014, June 7) Pot for pets? Cannabis now helping dogs and cats. Retrieved from the CNBC website.

2. Graulau, B. (2015, December 23) More using Cannabis-derived medication for their pets. Retrieved from the ABC10 website: http://www.abc10.com/news/more-using-cannabis-derived-medication-for-their-pets/22956968

APPENDIX I

PET OWNER SURVEY RESULTS

STUDIES SHOW
among pet owners with an opinion

The Department of Clinical Sciences at the Colorado State University College of Veterinary Medicine surveyed 457 dog owners via the Canna-Pet® website. Here are the results:

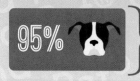

95% of dog owners felt that the consumption of hemp products **PROVIDED PAIN RELIEF** either moderately or a great deal.

- 92.6% favor Canna-Pet® to SOME, MOST OR ANY MEDICATIONS.

- 92% report Canna-Pet® helps RELIEVE SEIZURES OR CONVULSIONS a moderate amount or a lot.

- 78.6% report Canna-Pet® helps MUSCLE SPASMS a moderate amount or a lot.

- 70.8% report Canna-Pet® helps DIGESTIVE TRACT PROBLEMS a moderate amount or a lot.

- 73% report Canna-Pet® INHIBITED CELL GROWTH IN TUMORS a moderate amount or a lot.

- 61.8% report Canna-Pet® helps SKIN CONDITIONS a moderate amount or a lot.

- 88% report Canna-Pet® AIDS SLEEP a moderate amount or a lot.

- 91.9% report Canna-Pet® REDUCED INFLAMMATION a moderate amount or a lot.

- 82.3% report Canna-Pet® helps REDUCE VOMITING OR NAUSEA a moderate amount or a lot.

- 92.8% report Canna-Pet® provides NERVOUS SYSTEM SUPPORT a moderate amount or a lot.

83.2% of dog owners reported that hemp products HELPED RELIEVE ANXIETY either moderately or a great deal.

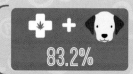

NATIONAL CANCER INSTITUTE

CANNABIS AND CANNABINOIDS (PDQ) — HEALTH PROFESSIONAL VERSION

Laboratory/Animal/Preclinical Studies
- **Antitumor Effects**
- **Antiemetic Effects**
- **Appetite Stimulation**
- **Analgesia**
- **Anxiety and Sleep**

Cannabinoids are a group of 21-carbon-containing terpenophenolic compounds produced uniquely by Cannabis species (e.g., Cannabis sativaL.).[1,2] These plant-derived compounds may be referred to as phytocannabinoids. Although delta-9-tetrahydrocannabinol (THC) is the primary psychoactive ingredient, other known compounds with biologic activity are cannabinol (CBN), cannabidiol (CBD), cannabichromene (CBC), cannabigerol (CBG), tetrahydrocannabivarin (THCV), and delta-8-THC. CBD, in particular, is thought to have significant analgesic, anti-inflammatory, and anxiolytic activity without the psychoactive effect (high) of delta-9-THC.

ANTITUMOR EFFECTS

One study in mice and rats suggested that cannabinoids may have a protective effect against the development of certain types of tumors.[3] During this 2-year study, groups of mice and rats were given various doses of THC by gavage. A dose-related decrease in the incidence of hepatic adenoma tumors and hepatocellular carcinoma (HCC) was observed in the mice. Decreased incidences of benign tumors (polyps and adenomas) in other organs (mammary gland, uterus, pituitary, testis, and pancreas) were also noted in the rats. In another study, delta-9-THC, delta-8-THC, and cannabinol were found to inhibit the growth of Lewis lung adenocarcinoma cells in vitro and in vivo.[4] In addition, other tumors have been shown to be sensitive to cannabinoid-induced growth inhibition.[5–8]

Cannabinoids may cause antitumor effects by various mechanisms, including induction of cell death, inhibition of cell growth, and inhibition of tumor angiogenesis invasion and metastasis.[9–12] Two reviews summarize the molecular mechanisms of action of cannabinoids as antitumor agents.[13,14] Cannabinoids appear to kill tumor cells but do not affect their nontransformed counterparts and may even protect them from cell death. For example, these compounds have been shown to induce apoptosis in glioma cells in culture and induce regression of glioma tumors in mice and rats, while they protect normal glial cells of astroglial and oligodendroglial lineages from apoptosis mediated by the CB1 receptor.[9]

The effects of delta-9-THC and a synthetic agonist of the CB2 receptor were investigated in HCC.[15] Both agents reduced the viability of HCC cells in vitro and demonstrated antitumor effects in HCC subcutaneous xenografts in nude mice. The investigations documented that the anti-HCC effects are mediated by way of the CB2 receptor. Similar to findings in glioma cells, the cannabinoids were shown to trigger cell death through stimulation of an endoplasmic reticulum stress pathway that activates autophagy and promotes apoptosis. Other investigations have confirmed that CB1 and CB2 receptors may be potential targets in non-small cell lung carcinoma[16] and breast cancer.[17]

An in vitro study of the effect of CBD on programmed cell death in breast cancer cell lines found that CBD induced programmed cell death, independent of the CB1, CB2, or vanilloid receptors. CBD inhibited the survival of both estrogen receptor-positive and estrogen receptor-negative breast cancer cell lines, inducing apoptosis in a concentration-dependent manner while having little effect on nontumorigenic mammary cells.[18] Other studies have also shown the antitumor effect of cannabinoids (i.e., CBD and THC) in preclinical models of breast cancer.[19,20]

CBD has also been demonstrated to exert a chemopreventive effect in a mouse model of colon cancer.[21] In this experimental system, azoxymethane increased premalignant and malignant lesions in the mouse colon. Animals treated with azoxymethane and CBD concurrently were protected from developing premalignant and malignant lesions. In in vitro experiments involving colorectal cancer cell lines, the investigators found that CBD protected DNA from oxidative damage, increased endocannabinoid levels, and reduced cell proliferation. In a subsequent study, the investigators found that the antiproliferative effect of CBD was counteracted by selective CB1 but not CB2 receptor antagonists, suggesting an involvement of CB1 receptors.[22]

Another investigation into the antitumor effects of CBD examined the role of intercellular adhesion molecule-1 (ICAM-1).[12] ICAM-1 expression has been reported to be negatively correlated with cancer metastasis. In lung cancer cell lines, CBD upregulated ICAM-1, leading to decreased cancer cell invasiveness.

In an in vivo model using severe combined immunodeficient mice, subcutaneous tumors were generated by inoculating the animals with cells from human non-small cell lung carcinoma cell lines.[23] Tumor growth was inhibited by 60% in THC-treated mice compared with vehicle-treated control mice. Tumor specimens revealed that THC had antiangiogenic and antiproliferative effects. However, research with immunocompetent murine tumor models has demonstrated immunosuppression and enhanced tumor growth in mice treated with THC.[24,25]

In addition, both plant-derived and endogenous cannabinoids have been studied for anti-inflammatory effects. A mouse study demonstrated that endogenous cannabinoid system signaling is likely to provide intrinsic protection against colonic inflammation.[26] As a result, a hypothesis that phytocannabinoids and endocannabinoids may be useful in the risk reduction and treatment of colorectal cancer has been developed.[27–30]

CBD may also enhance uptake of cytotoxic drugs into malignant cells. Activation of the transient receptor potential vanilloid type 2 (TRPV2) has been shown to inhibit proliferation of human glioblastoma multiforme cells and overcome resistance to the chemotherapy agent carmustine.[31] One study showed that coadministration of THC and CBD over single-agent usage had greater antiproliferative activity in an in vitro study with multiple human glioblastoma multiforme cell lines.[32] In an in vitro model, CBD increased TRPV2 activation and increased uptake of cytotoxic drugs, leading to apoptosis of glioma cells without affecting normal human astrocytes. This suggests that coadministration of CBD with cytotoxic agents may increase drug uptake and potentiate cell death in human glioma cells. Also, CBD together with THC may enhance the antitumor activity of classic chemotherapeutic drugs such as temozolomide in some mouse models of cancer.[13,33]

ANTIEMETIC EFFECTS

Preclinical research suggests that emetic circuitry is tonically controlled by endocannabinoids. The antiemetic action of cannabinoids is believed to be mediated via interaction with the 5-hydroxytryptamine 3 (5-HT3) receptor. CB1 receptors and 5-HT3 receptors are colocalized on gamma-aminobutyric acid (GABA)-ergic neurons, where they have opposite effects on GABA release.[34] There also may be direct inhibition of 5-HT3 gated ion currents through non-CB1 receptor pathways. CB1 receptor antagonists have been shown to elicit emesis in the least shrew that is reversed by cannabinoid agonists.[35] The involvement of CB1 receptor in emesis prevention has been shown by the ability of CB1 antagonists to reverse the effects of THC and other synthetic cannabinoid CB1 agonists in suppressing vomiting caused by cisplatin in the house musk shrew and lithium chloride in the least shrew. In the latter model, CBD was also shown to be efficacious.[36,37]

APPETITE STIMULATION

Many animal studies have previously demonstrated that delta-9-THC and other cannabinoids have a stimulatory effect on appetite and increase food intake. It is believed that the endogenous cannabinoid system may serve as a regulator of feeding behavior. The endogenous cannabinoid anandamide potently enhances appetite in mice.[38] Moreover, CB1 receptors in the hypothalamus may be involved in the motivational or reward aspects of eating.[39]

ANALGESIA

Understanding the mechanism of cannabinoid-induced analgesia has been increased through the study of cannabinoid receptors, endocannabinoids, and synthetic agonists and antagonists. Cannabinoids produce analgesia through supraspinal, spinal, and peripheral modes of action, acting on both ascending and descending pain pathways.[40] The CB1 receptor is found in both the central nervous system (CNS) and in peripheral nerve terminals. Similar to opioid receptors, increased levels of the CB1 receptor are found in regions of the brain that regulate nociceptive processing.[41] CB2 receptors, located predominantly in peripheral tissue, exist at very low levels in the CNS. With the development of receptor-specific antagonists, additional information about the roles of the receptors and endogenous cannabinoids in the modulation of pain has been obtained.[42,43]

Cannabinoids may also contribute to pain modulation through an anti-inflammatory mechanism; a CB2 effect with cannabinoids acting on mast cell receptors to attenuate the release of inflammatory agents, such as histamine and serotonin, and on keratinocytes to enhance the release of analgesic opioids has been described.[44–46] One study reported that the efficacy of synthetic CB1- and CB2-receptor agonists were comparable with the efficacy of morphine in a murine model of tumor pain.[47]

Cannabinoids have been shown to prevent chemotherapy-induced neuropathy in animal models exposed to paclitaxel, vincristine, or cisplatin.[48–50]

ANXIETY AND SLEEP

The endocannabinoid system is believed to be centrally involved in the regulation of mood and the extinction of aversive memories. Animal studies have shown CBD to have anxiolytic properties. It was shown in rats that these anxiolytic properties are mediated through unknown mechanisms.[51] Anxiolytic effects of CBD have been shown in several animal models.[52,53]

The endocannabinoid system has also been shown to play a key role in the modulation of the sleep-waking cycle in rats.[54,55]

REFERENCES

1. Adams IB, Martin BR: Cannabis: pharmacology and toxicology in animals and humans. Addiction 91 (11): 1585-614, 1996. [PUBMED Abstract]

2. Grotenhermen F, Russo E, eds.: Cannabis and Cannabinoids: Pharmacology, Toxicology, and Therapeutic Potential. Binghamton, NY: The Haworth Press, 2002.

3. National Toxicology Program: NTP toxicology and carcinogenesis studies of 1-transdelta(9)-tetrahydrocannabinol (CAS No. 1972-08-3) in F344 rats and B6C3F1 mice (gavage studies). Natl Toxicol Program Tech Rep Ser 446 (): 1-317, 1996. [PUBMED Abstract]

4. Bifulco M, Laezza C, Pisanti S, et al.: Cannabinoids and cancer: pros and cons of an antitumour strategy. Br J Pharmacol 148 (2): 123-35, 2006. [PUBMED Abstract]

5. Sánchez C, de Ceballos ML, Gomez del Pulgar T, et al.: Inhibition of glioma growth in vivo by selective activation of the CB(2) cannabinoid receptor. Cancer Res 61 (15): 5784-9, 2001. [PUBMED Abstract]

6. McKallip RJ, Lombard C, Fisher M, et al.: Targeting CB2 cannabinoid receptors as a novel therapy to treat malignant lymphoblastic disease. Blood 100 (2): 627-34, 2002. [PUBMED Abstract]

7. Casanova ML, Blázquez C, Martínez-Palacio J, et al.: Inhibition of skin tumor growth and angiogenesis in vivo by activation of cannabinoid receptors. J Clin Invest 111 (1): 43-50, 2003. [PUBMED Abstract]

8. Blázquez C, González-Feria L, Alvarez L, et al.: Cannabinoids inhibit the vascular endothelial growth factor pathway in gliomas. Cancer Res 64 (16): 5617-23, 2004. [PUBMED Abstract]

9. Guzmán M: Cannabinoids: potential anticancer agents. Nat Rev Cancer 3 (10): 745-55, 2003. [PUBMED Abstract]

10. Blázquez C, Casanova ML, Planas A, et al.: Inhibition of tumor angiogenesis by cannabinoids. FASEB J 17 (3): 529-31, 2003. [PUBMED Abstract]

11. Vaccani A, Massi P, Colombo A, et al.: Cannabidiol inhibits human glioma cell migration through a cannabinoid receptor-independent mechanism. Br J Pharmacol 144 (8): 1032-6, 2005. [PUBMED Abstract]

12. Ramer R, Bublitz K, Freimuth N, et al.: Cannabidiol inhibits lung cancer cell invasion and metastasis via intercellular adhesion molecule-1. FASEB J 26 (4): 1535-48, 2012. [PUBMED Abstract]

13. Velasco G, Sánchez C, Guzmán M: Towards the use of cannabinoids as antitumour agents. Nat Rev Cancer 12 (6): 436-44, 2012. [PUBMED Abstract]

14. Cridge BJ, Rosengren RJ: Critical appraisal of the potential use of cannabinoids in cancer management. Cancer Manag Res 5: 301-13, 2013. [PUBMED Abstract]

15. Vara D, Salazar M, Olea-Herrero N, et al.: Anti-tumoral action of cannabinoids on hepatocellular carcinoma: role of AMPK-dependent activation of autophagy. Cell Death Differ 18 (7): 1099-111, 2011. [PUBMED Abstract]

16. Preet A, Qamri Z, Nasser MW, et al.: Cannabinoid receptors, CB1 and CB2, as novel targets for inhibition of non-small cell lung cancer growth and metastasis. Cancer Prev Res (Phila) 4(1): 65-75, 2011. [PUBMED Abstract]

17. Nasser MW, Qamri Z, Deol YS, et al.: Crosstalk between chemokine receptor CXCR4 and cannabinoid receptor CB2 in modulating breast cancer growth and invasion. PLoS One 6 (9): e23901, 2011. [PUBMED Abstract]

18. Shrivastava A, Kuzontkoski PM, Groopman JE, et al.: Cannabidiol induces programmed cell death in breast cancer cells by coordinating the cross-talk between apoptosis and autophagy. Mol Cancer Ther 10 (7): 1161-72, 2011. [PUBMED Abstract]

19. Caffarel MM, Andradas C, Mira E, et al.: Cannabinoids reduce ErbB2-driven breast cancer progression through Akt inhibition. Mol Cancer 9: 196, 2010. [PUBMED Abstract]

20. McAllister SD, Murase R, Christian RT, et al.: Pathways mediating the effects of cannabidiol on the reduction of breast cancer cell proliferation, invasion, and metastasis. Breast Cancer Res Treat 129 (1): 37-47, 2011. [PUBMED Abstract]

21. Aviello G, Romano B, Borrelli F, et al.: Chemopreventive effect of the non-psychotropic phytocannabinoid cannabidiol on experimental colon cancer. J Mol Med (Berl) 90 (8): 925-34, 2012. [PUBMED Abstract]

22. Romano B, Borrelli F, Pagano E, et al.: Inhibition of colon carcinogenesis by a standardized Cannabis sativa extract with high content of cannabidiol. Phytomedicine 21 (5): 631-9, 2014. [PUBMED Abstract]

23. Preet A, Ganju RK, Groopman JE: Delta9-Tetrahydrocannabinol inhibits epithelial growth factor-induced lung cancer cell migration in vitro as well as its growth and metastasis in vivo. Oncogene 27 (3): 339-46, 2008. [PUBMED Abstract]

24. Zhu LX, Sharma S, Stolina M, et al.: Delta-9-tetrahydrocannabinol inhibits antitumor immunity by a CB2 receptor-mediated, cytokine-dependent pathway. J Immunol 165 (1): 373-80, 2000. [PUBMED Abstract]

25. McKallip RJ, Nagarkatti M, Nagarkatti PS: Delta-9-tetrahydrocannabinol enhances breast cancer growth and metastasis by suppression of the antitumor immune response. J Immunol 174 (6): 3281-9, 2005. [PUBMED Abstract]

26. Massa F, Marsicano G, Hermann H, et al.: The endogenous cannabinoid system protects against colonic inflammation. J Clin Invest 113 (8): 1202-9, 2004. [PUBMED Abstract]

27. Patsos HA, Hicks DJ, Greenhough A, et al.: Cannabinoids and cancer: potential for colorectal cancer therapy. Biochem Soc Trans 33 (Pt 4): 712-4, 2005. [PUBMED Abstract]

28. Liu WM, Fowler DW, Dalgleish AG: Cannabis-derived substances in cancer therapy—an emerging anti-inflammatory role for the cannabinoids. Curr Clin Pharmacol 5 (4): 281-7, 2010. [PUBMED Abstract]

29. Malfitano AM, Ciaglia E, Gangemi G, et al.: Update on the endocannabinoid system as an anticancer target. Expert Opin Ther Targets 15 (3): 297-308, 2011. [PUBMED Abstract]

30. Sarfaraz S, Adhami VM, Syed DN, et al.: Cannabinoids for cancer treatment: progress and promise. Cancer Res 68 (2): 339-42, 2008. [PUBMED Abstract]

31. Nabissi M, Morelli MB, Santoni M, et al.: Triggering of the TRPV2 channel by cannabidiol sensitizes glioblastoma cells to cytotoxic chemotherapeutic agents. Carcinogenesis 34 (1): 48-57, 2013. [PUBMED Abstract]

32. Marcu JP, Christian RT, Lau D, et al.: Cannabidiol enhances the inhibitory effects of delta9-tetrahydrocannabinol on human glioblastoma cell

proliferation and survival. Mol Cancer Ther 9 (1): 180-9, 2010. [PUBMED Abstract]

33. Torres S, Lorente M, Rodríguez-Fornés F, et al.: A combined preclinical therapy of cannabinoids and temozolomide against glioma. Mol Cancer Ther 10 (1): 90-103, 2011. [PUBMED Abstract]

34. Pacher P, Bátkai S, Kunos G: The endocannabinoid system as an emerging target of pharmacotherapy. Pharmacol Rev 58 (3): 389-462, 2006. [PUBMED Abstract]

35. Darmani NA: Delta(9)-tetrahydrocannabinol and synthetic cannabinoids prevent emesis produced by the cannabinoid CB(1) receptor antagonist/inverse agonist SR 141716A. Neuropsychopharmacology 24 (2): 198-203, 2001. [PUBMED Abstract]

36. Darmani NA: Delta-9-tetrahydrocannabinol differentially suppresses cisplatin-induced emesis and indices of motor function via cannabinoid CB(1) receptors in the least shrew. Pharmacol Biochem Behav 69 (1-2): 239-49, 2001 May-Jun. [PUBMED Abstract]

37. Parker LA, Kwiatkowska M, Burton P, et al.: Effect of cannabinoids on lithium-induced vomiting in the Suncus murinus (house musk shrew). Psychopharmacology (Berl) 171 (2): 156-61, 2004. [PUBMED Abstract]

38. Mechoulam R, Berry EM, Avraham Y, et al.: Endocannabinoids, feeding and suckling—from our perspective. Int J Obes (Lond) 30 (Suppl 1): S24-8, 2006. [PUBMED Abstract]

39. Fride E, Bregman T, Kirkham TC: Endocannabinoids and food intake: newborn suckling and appetite regulation in adulthood. Exp Biol Med (Maywood) 230 (4): 225-34, 2005. [PUBMED Abstract]

40. Baker D, Pryce G, Giovannoni G, et al.: The therapeutic potential of cannabis. Lancet Neurol 2(5): 291-8, 2003. [PUBMED Abstract]

41. Walker JM, Hohmann AG, Martin WJ, et al.: The neurobiology of cannabinoid analgesia. Life Sci 65 (6-7): 665-73, 1999. [PUBMED Abstract]

42. Meng ID, Manning BH, Martin WJ, et al.: An analgesia circuit activated by cannabinoids. Nature 395 (6700): 381-3, 1998. [PUBMED Abstract]

43. Walker JM, Huang SM, Strangman NM, et al.: Pain modulation by release of the endogenous cannabinoid anandamide. Proc Natl Acad Sci USA 96 (21): 12198-203, 1999. [PUBMED Abstract]

44. Facci L, Dal Toso R, Romanello S, et al.: Mast cells express a peripheral cannabinoid receptor with differential sensitivity to anandamide and palmitoylethanolamide. Proc Natl Acad Sci USA 92 (8): 3376-80, 1995. [PUBMED Abstract]

45. Ibrahim MM, Porreca F, Lai J, et al.: CB2 cannabinoid receptor activation produces antinociception by stimulating peripheral release of endogenous opioids. Proc Natl Acad Sci USA 102 (8): 3093-8, 2005. [PUBMED Abstract]

46. Richardson JD, Kilo S, Hargreaves KM: Cannabinoids reduce hyperalgesia and inflammation via interaction with peripheral CB1 receptors. Pain 75 (1): 111-9, 1998. [PUBMED Abstract]

47. Khasabova IA, Gielissen J, Chandiramani A, et al.: CB1 and CB2 receptor agonists promote analgesia through synergy in a murine model of tumor pain. Behav Pharmacol 22 (5-6): 607-16, 2011. [PUBMED Abstract]

48. Ward SJ, McAllister SD, Kawamura R, et al.: Cannabidiol inhibits paclitaxel-induced neuropathic pain through 5-HT(1A) receptors without diminishing nervous system function or chemotherapy efficacy. Br J Pharmacol 171 (3): 636-45, 2014. [PUBMED Abstract]

49. Rahn EJ, Makriyannis A, Hohmann AG: Activation of cannabinoid CB1 and CB2 receptors suppresses neuropathic nociception evoked by the chemotherapeutic agent vincristine in rats. Br J Pharmacol 152 (5): 765-77, 2007. [PUBMED Abstract]

50. Khasabova IA, Khasabov S, Paz J, et al.: Cannabinoid type-1 receptor reduces pain and neurotoxicity produced by chemotherapy. J Neurosci 32 (20): 7091-101, 2012. [PUBMED Abstract]

51. Campos AC, Guimarães FS: Involvement of 5HT1A receptors in the anxiolytic-like effects of cannabidiol injected into the dorsolateral periaqueductal gray of rats. Psychopharmacology (Berl) 199 (2): 223-30, 2008. [PUBMED Abstract]

52. Crippa JA, Zuardi AW, Hallak JE: [Therapeutical use of the cannabinoids in psychiatry]. Rev Bras Psiquiatr 32 (Suppl 1): S56-66, 2010. [PUBMED Abstract]

53. Guimarães FS, Chiaretti TM, Graeff FG, et al.: Antianxiety effect of cannabidiol in the elevated plus-maze. Psychopharmacology (Berl) 100 (4): 558-9, 1990. [PUBMED Abstract]

54. Méndez-Díaz M, Caynas-Rojas S, Arteaga Santacruz V, et al.: Entope-duncular nucleus endocannabinoid system modulates sleep-waking cycle and mood in rats. Pharmacol Biochem Behav 107: 29-35, 2013. [PUBMED Abstract]

55. Pava MJ, den Hartog CR, Blanco-Centurion C, et al.: Endocannabinoid modulation of cortical up-states and NREM sleep. PLoS One 9 (2): e88672, 2014. [PUBMED Abstract]

APPENDIX III

PHYTOCANNABINOID-TERPENOID ENTOURAGE EFFECTS

BRITISH JOURNAL OF PHARMACOLOGY

Table 1

Phytocannabinoid activity table

Phytocannabinoid structure	Selected pharmacology (reference)	Synergistic terpenoids
delta-9-tetrahydrocannabinol (THC)	Analgesic via CB_1 and CB_2 (Rahn and Hohmann, 2009)	Various
	AI/antioxidant (Hampson et al., 1998)	Limonene et al.
	Bronchodilatory (Williams et al., 1976)	Pinene
	↓ Sx. Alzheimer disease (Volicer et al., 1997; Eubanks et al., 2006)	Limonene, pinene, linalool
	Benefit on duodenal ulcers (Douthwaite, 1947)	Caryophyllene, limonene
	Muscle relaxant (Kavia et al., 2010)	Linalool?
	Antipruritic, cholestatic jaundice (Neff et al., 2002)	Caryophyllene?
cannabidiol	AI/antioxidant (Hampson et al., 1998)	Limonene et al.
	Anti-anxiety via $5-HT_{1A}$ (Russo et al., 2005)	Linalool, limonene
	Anticonvulsant (Jones et al., 2010)	Linalool
	Cytotoxic versus breast cancer (Ligresti et al., 2006)	Limonene
	↑ adenosine A_{2A} signalling (Carrier et al., 2006)	Linalool
	Effective versus MRSA (Appendino et al., 2008)	Pinene
	Decreases sebum/sebocytes (Biro et al., 2009)	Pinene, limonene, linalool
	Treatment of addiction (see text)	Caryophyllene
cannabichromene	Anti-inflammatory/analgesic (Davis and Hatoum, 1983)	Various
	Antifungal (ElSohly et al., 1982)	Caryophyllene oxide
	AEA uptake inhibitor (De Petrocellis et al., 2011)	–
	Antidepressant in rodent model (Deyo and Musty, 2003)	Limonene
cannabigerol	TRPM8 antagonist prostate cancer (De Petrocellis et al., 2011)	Cannabis terpenoids
	GABA uptake inhibitor (Banerjee et al., 1975)	Phytol, linalool
	Anti-fungal (ElSohly et al., 1982)	Caryophyllene oxide
	Antidepressant rodent model (Musty and Deyo, 2006); and via $5-HT_{1A}$ antagonism (Cascio et al., 2010)	Limonene
	Analgesic, α-2 adrenergic blockade (Cascio et al., 2010)	Various
	↓ keratinocytes in psoriasis (Wilkinson and Williamson, 2007)	adjunctive role?
	Effective versus MRSA (Appendino et al., 2008)	Pinene
tetrahydrocannabivarin	AI/anti-hyperalgesic (Bolognini et al., 2010)	Caryophyllene et al. . . .
	Treatment of metabolic syndrome (Cawthorne et al., 2007)	–
	Anticonvulsant (Hill et al., 2010)	Linalool
cannabidivarin	Inhibits diacylglycerol lipase (De Petrocellis et al., 2011)	–
	Anticonvulsant in hippocampus (Hill et al., 2010)	Linalool
cannabinol (CBN)	Sedative (Musty et al., 1976)	Nerolidol, myrcene
	Effective versus MRSA (Appendino et al., 2008)	Pinene
	TRPV2 agonist for burns (Qin et al., 2008)	Linalool
	↓ keratinocytes in psoriasis (Wilkinson and Williamson, 2007)	adjunctive role?
	↓ breast cancer resistance protein (Holland et al., 2008)	Limonene

5-HT, 5-hydroxytryptamine (serotonin); AEA, arachidonoylethanolamide (anandamide); AI, anti-inflammatory; CB1/CB2, cannabinoid receptor 1 or 2; GABA, gamma aminobutyric acid; TRPV, transient receptor potential vanilloid receptor; MRSA, methicillin-resistant *Staphylococcus aureus*; Sx, symptoms.

Phytocannabinoid-terpenoid entourage effects

Table 2
Cannabis Terpenoid Activity Table

Terpenoid	Structure	Commonly encountered in	Pharmacological activity (Reference)	Synergistic cannabinoid
Limonene		Lemon	Potent AD/immunostimulant via inhalation (Komori et al., 1995)	CBD
			Anxiolytic (Carvalho-Freitas and Costa, 2002; Pultrini Ade et al., 2006) via 5-HT₁A (Komiya et al., 2006)	CBD
			Apoptosis of breast cancer cells (Vigushin et al., 1998)	CBD, CBG
			Active against acne bacteria (Kim et al., 2008)	CBD
			Dermatophytes (Sanguinetti et al., 2007; Singh et al., 2010)	CBG
			Gastro-oesophageal reflux (Harris, 2010)	THC
α-Pinene		Pine	Anti-inflammatory via PGE-1 (Gil et al., 1989)	CBD
			Bronchodilatory in humans (Falk et al., 1990)	THC
			Acetylcholinesterase inhibitor, aiding memory (Perry et al., 2000)	THC?, CBD
β-Myrcene		Hops	Blocks inflammation via PGE-2 (Lorenzetti et al., 1991)	CBD
			Analgesic, antagonized by naloxone (Rao et al., 1990)	CBD, THC
			Sedating, muscle relaxant, hypnotic (do Vale et al., 2002)	THC
			Blocks hepatic carcinogenesis by aflatoxin (de Oliveira et al., 1997)	CBD, CBG
Linalool		Lavender	Anti-anxiety (Russo, 2001)	CBD, CBG?
			Sedative on inhalation in mice (Buchbauer et al., 1993)	THC
			Local anesthetic (Re et al., 2000)	THC
			Analgesic via adenosine A₂A (Peana et al., 2006)	CBD
			Anticonvulsant/anti-glutamate (Elisabetsky et al., 1995)	CBD, THCV, CBDV
			Potent anti-leishmanial (do Socorro et al., 2003)	?
β-Caryophyllene		Pepper	AI via PGE-1 comparable phenylbutazone (Basile et al., 1988)	CBD
			Gastric cytoprotective (Tambe et al., 1996)	THC
			Anti-malarial (Campbell et al., 1997)	?
			Selective CB₂ agonist (100 nM) (Gertsch et al., 2008)	THC
			Treatment of pruritus? (Karsak et al., 2007)	THC
			Treatment of addiction? (Xi et al., 2010)	CBD
Caryophyllene Oxide		Lemon balm	Decreases platelet aggregation (Lin et al., 2003)	THC
			Antifungal in onychomycosis comparable to ciclopiroxolamine and sulconazole (Yang et al., 1999)	CBC,CBG
			Insecticidal/anti-feedant (Bettarini et al., 1993)	THCA, CBGA
Nerolidol		Orange	Sedative (Binet et al., 1972)	THC, CBN
			Skin penetrant (Cornwell and Barry, 1994)	–
			Potent antimalarial (Lopes et al., 1999, Rodrigues Goulart et al., 2004)	?
			Anti-leishmanial activity (Arruda et al., 2005)	?
Phytol		Green tea	Breakdown product of chlorophyll	–
			Prevents Vitamin A teratogenesis (Arnhold et al., 2002)	–
			↑GABA via SSADH inhibition (Bang et al., 2002)	CBG

Representative plants containing each terpenoid are displayed as examples to promote recognition, but many species contain them in varying concentrations. 5-HT, 5-hydroxytryptamine (serotonin); AD, antidepressant; AI, anti-inflammatory; CB₁/CB₂, cannabinoid receptor 1 or 2; GABA, gamma aminobutyric acid; PGE-1/PGE-2, prostaglandin E-1/prostaglandin E-2; SSADH, succinic semialdehyde dehydrogenase.

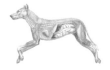

AUTHOR PROFILE

D. CAROLINE COILE, PH.D., has written 34 books and more than a thousand magazine and scientific articles about dogs and cats. Her books have sold more than a million copies, and include the top-selling dog breed encyclopedia, *Barron's Encyclopedia of Dog Breeds.* She wrote monthly columns for *Dog World* magazine and the *AKC Gazette* for more than a decade and currently writes regular columns for *AKC Family Dog* and *Show Sight* magazines, plus a weekly breed feature for Dogster.com.

She has been inducted in the Dog Writers Association of America Hall of Fame; other writing awards include the Dog Writers Association of America Maxwell Award (eight times), the DWAA Denlinger Award, the AKC Canine Health Foundation Research Communication Award (twice), the Eukanuba Canine Health Award (twice) and the Morris Animal Foundation Award.

Caroline holds a Ph.D. in Psychology from Florida State University, with research interests in canine behavior, senses, genetics and neuropsychology. She has taught college classes in biological psychology, animal senses, and animal learning, among others. She has served as a canine consultant to the FAA and the AKC Canine Health Foundation President's Counsel.

On a practical level, Caroline has lived with dogs all of her life. She shares her home with five salukis and one sort-of-Jack-Russell-if-you-squint—all of which help out by jumping on the keyboard before she manages to hit Save. Second drafts are always better anyway.